Freedom from Rheumatoid Arthritis

Freedom from Rheumatoid Arthritis

The amazing story of one woman's recovery

SONIA ST. CLAIRE

Let food be your medicine and medicine be your food
Hippocrates

Copyright © 2008 by Sonia St. Claire.

Library of Congress Control Number: 2008901366
ISBN: Hardcover 978-1-4363-2278-2
Softcover 978-1-4363-2277-5

All rights reserved. No part of this publication may be reproduced or transmitted in any form or by any means, mechanical or electronic, including photocopying and recording, or by any information storage and retrieval system, without permission in writing from the author.

DISCLAIMER

The opinions expressed in this book, unless otherwise attributed, are those of the author Sonia St. Claire.

The Author neither makes nor attempts to make any diagnosis or cure or prevent any disease. The author will not accept any responsibility for any loss, injury or damage caused or allegedly caused, directly or indirectly by the information contained in this book. The purpose of this book is to share my story and information I have acquired over the years. It is your choice to follow any or all of this information. If unsure, please check with your health care professional

This way of eating helped me to overcome rheumatoid arthritis and it may help you.

PERMISSIONS

The Health Revolution and *Improving on Pritikin*
Ross Horne

Total Health
Dr. Joseph Mercola
Wayne Beamer (Mercola.com)

This book was printed in the United States of America.

To order additional copies of this book, contact:
Xlibris Corporation
1-888-795-4274
www.Xlibris.com
Orders@Xlibris.com
47817

CONTENTS

Chapter 1   In the Beginning 15

Chapter 2   Testing Times 35

Chapter 3   Root Causes 40

Chapter 4   Where Death Begins 46

Chapter 5   Natural Solutions 56

Chapter 6   Recovery in Context 63

Chapter 7   Recovery Diet 84

Chapter 8   Recovery diet 7 day menu 94

Chapter 9   Recipes Recovery Diet 107

Chapter 10   Recipes Maintenance diet 129

Chapter 11   Raw/vegan diet 149

Conclusion 157

Bibliography 173

DEDICATION

I dedicate this book to all the sufferers of rheumatoid arthritis, including the souls who took their own lives due to the unrelenting chronic pain they could no longer endure. My thoughts are with you.

Acknowledgements

My sincere love, appreciation and thanks go to my son Ben and my daughter Olivia. Without their love and support during my time of illness when I was lost in my world, I don't know what I would have done, or how I would have ended up. They cared about what hurt me. They gave me the courage to go on. I am forever grateful and privileged to have them both in my life. I am honored to be their mother.

Without their help I may not have discovered myself. The ultimate person I can be. Young children have an extraordinary way of looking at the world. They stepped up and delivered without question, with love in their hearts and innocence in their eyes.

Furthermore, I want to take this opportunity to remind them, what they all ready know is true, 'I love them.' They brought me sustainable joy, bliss and happiness. I have treasured every moment raising them and the memories of their innocence during their primary years, are locked away in my heart forever.

In Appreciation

To Miriam, I want to thank you for always believing in me, and the success of this book. Your support is greatly appreciated.

To Steve, your support is also greatly appreciated. Thank you.

Thank you to Joan for your generosity.

Thank you to Lorraine for taking my photo for this book.

I can be contacted through my website address *www.ffra.com*

I have a dream

Martin Luther King Jr.
August 28, 1963

Our life is what our thoughts make it

Marcus Aurelius Antonius

People only see what they are prepared to see
Ralph Waldo Emerson

We don't see things as they are; we see them as we are
Anais Nin

Chapter 1

—*In the beginning*—

Compassion for humanity is my motivation in writing this book. For it is their suffering—of this dreadful disease that compels me to make people aware that, there is a way to bring about a natural remission of Rheumatoid Arthritis (R.A An auto-immune disease that attacks the body's own defense system.) A natural remission can occur when the body is fed proper nutrition. I know this to be true from my own personal experience. My personal encounter is the wellspring of the compassion that motivates the desire to share my story. Compassion provided the force and energy for me to try to make people aware that there is a way of achieving a natural remission.

It was May 1994. One month before my forty-fourth birthday when I was diagnosed with the condition known as rheumatoid arthritis (RA). For me the onset of this disease was slow. I simply felt unwell for a long time. During the years that I suffered from RA, I learned the hard way about what was healthy for me, and what was not. My willingness to spend hundreds of dollars, parting with what little money I had, was a reflection of my despair over the agony I was suffering from this insidious disease. I tried just about everything there was on the market, but nothing helped. I was vulnerable and on the verge of suicide.

Being ill and in such deep despair taught me many lessons. I learned there are some unscrupulous people who are willing to prey on the ailing. In fact, I discovered during my illness that you almost allow yourself to fall victim to such people who see the ill as easy prey. I learned that being ill meant you were at the bottom rung of the ladder of society. I also learned there was even a form of snobbery amongst the different disabilities that determined ranking and treatment within the health system. I realized being an ill person was not the person I wanted to be.

I never saw myself before in this way, an ill person with no credibility, a person of no value in society. I had never imagined myself the way others now saw me. I had to introduce myself to the person whom I had become, because I could no longer remember the person I used to be. Because of my ailing health, I realized I could no longer choose who I am. I had to try to remember the person I was supposed to be.

At this particular time in my life, the thought of ending it all to relieve my anguish would have been a welcome relief. Unless you have been afflicted with this hideous disease you could not know, you could not understand, nor, could you appreciate the chronic, unyielding pain. It is only if you have the misfortune to experience an illness such as this that you realize the depths of torment and sorrow it brings. I refused to give up and continued to live in hope. I therefore continued to use what little resources I had on natural lotions, potions, vitamins and just about every arthritis cream available because the chronic pain from my body almost drove my mind insane. The only natural product that gave me some kind of relief in reducing my pain level was Zinaxin joint care, a natural ginger I found in my local health food store and chemist. Or perhaps you could try fresh ginger in your juices. Due to the chemical components and horrific side effects (diseases brought on by the body from the medication) on the body, I prefer natural products as opposed to drug therapy.

I was, in fact, much more afraid of the drug therapy than the disease itself and refused to take chemical prescription drugs. One rheumatologist told me if I did not take the prescribed rheumatic drugs, I would end up a useless cripple, wheelchair bound and would not be able to use my hands to dress myself. He also became cross with me when I refused to accept his prescription. Because of his bullying behavior toward me, I found myself another rheumatologist who proved to be a charming, mild mannered and gentle man whom I held in high esteem. When he suggested that I at least try drug therapy, I surrendered, even though my intuition said no.

The first medication to be tried was Methotrexate, a chemotherapy drug that is often prescribed for RA sufferers. I was on this medication for six weeks when I decided to stop taking it due to abdominal pain and diarrhea which necessitated a colonoscopy. The results was in fact, drug induced colitis. Next, I tried Salazopyren. This drug resulted in me feeling like a zombie with the sensation of a head too big for my body. I could barely function. It seemed that I was ready to topple over at any moment.

Because of taking this particular drug, I spent most of my time on the lounge, unwell and virtually incoherent; it was increasingly difficult to comprehend what people were saying to me. I was in a perpetual mental fog and detached from my own body and, again, after six weeks I took myself off the medication. I tried the non-steroidal anti-inflammatory drugs and 500mg tablets of Panamax pain killers. In addition, I tried Prednisolone and was not even aware at the time of cortisone's deadly side effects. I refused, however, to have gold injections. I was, in short, a walking chemistry lab. (However, I was never on Vioxx. This drug in October 2004 was discovered to double your risk of heart attack and stroke and has caused deaths. Vioxx has been recalled world wide. My intuition was telling me not to take the drugs and I was right. I was told that RA was incurable, that insidious deformities would occur, and the only way to slow down the pace of the disease was through drug therapy. I asked whether the disease would go into remission on medication and was told by my doctor that drug induced remission was possible. However, this would only last for about a year as RA had a way of showing up elsewhere in the body. In other words, the drugs mask the disease; they do not affect a cure. I would, in consequence, have to not only endure the arthritis but also the hideous side effects brought on by the medication. To me this was tantamount to dealing with two diseases and I was exhausted by the struggle to deal with just one. Already in a deep depression over the loss of my health, I really did not care whether I lived or died. The disease and the chronic pain it caused me had turned my life into a prison sentence to be endured, with no prospect of a cure. I was not living my life now; I merely existed as I breathed in and out and tried to stay alive for my children.

I wanted to make my life have a purpose, to live beyond just existing. I wanted to rise from this disease and live as if I had never lived before. Under the influence of great emotion and distress my life now lacked significance caught up as I was in the terror of my daily torment and a future that appeared even bleaker. Over time my hands became very painful, especially the palms of my hands and several of the finger joints. Splints designed to help only caused my hands to become stiffer. I swallowed as many painkillers as permitted although there were many days when I took double the dose.

My days passed in a fog of pain and lethargy mostly on the lounge, in front of the television. One of the most insidious aspects of RA is that it prevents the body from accessing iron with the result that chronic anemia becomes part of the disease. If it were not for my son Ben, and my daughter Olivia, who were only eight and six years of age, respectively, at the time, I do not know how I would have coped. With no extended family to call upon for help, the children were fast becoming efficient in the kitchen and learned to fend for themselves. To reach out to strangers was not in my make-up, therefore, on my really bad days my children did not go to school and, especially when I became bedridden, both Ben and Olivia stayed home to look after me. During this time, they dressed, fed and bathed me. They brushed my hair and told me they loved me. When I needed to get out of bed to go to the bathroom, my children sat me in the upright position and turned my body around so my feet touched the floor. Then, they pulled me off the bed, shuffled me into the toilet, sat me on the bowl and left me in privacy. There I sat, trying to fight for every single day. They waited like "loyal angels" then pulled me up and pushed me along into the shower. To hold or turn a tap was now utterly beyond me. My eight year-old little boy ran the water. My natural strength had deserted me. My mind and body cringed at the indignities imposed by being chronically ill.

I stood naked and helpless as the shower water flowed over my agonizingly painful body, merging with my tears as I attempted to get through the day. Holding onto the shower wall, I pondered on my life; the misery set before me each day; the intolerable pain that ate away at my soul. It was my children and only my children who kept me on the earth that savaged me so much. For them I had to endure my life, and wrap myself in God's will and exist for them. For me, however, my existence was measured by pain and anguish and its bleakness frightened me.

My children also suffered because they no longer had an able-bodied mother who took care of them. They now had a mother who was chronically ill, in constant pain and under the influence of great emotion. Tears and anguish had replaced the laughter and mobility I once knew. The disease had changed me, totally. In being unable to do even the simplest tasks, I became depressed and resentful. I could no longer put Olivia's hair into a ponytail or braids. It was agonizing just to hold the hairbrush in my hands and to place my thumb and forefinger together was excruciating.

On and off for a year and a half during the time I was bedridden, the children were left unsupervised in the kitchen. It became their domain. They ate whatever they could out of a packet or can. They were under strict instructions not to use the stove in case they set fire to themselves and the house. The kettle and the toaster were permitted to be used. They made me cups of tea and toast for breakfast, spaghetti sandwiches for lunch and cereal for dinner. I could not believe what I saw when, after several days of my first experience in a bedridden condition, I crawled along the wall and out into the kitchen. The kitchen bench and floor were strewn with litter, empty packets and cans. The place looked like the local tip. I burst into tears—not because the kitchen was dirty, but because my young children were forced to take care of themselves.

However, in the face of my misery, their faces told a different story. They were happy and excited to see me, and proud of looking after me and doing such a fine job. Their innocence touched me. They occupied themselves tending to me, oblivious to the untidiness of the house; I was swept up in the spirit of my children; it was beautiful.

I phoned home help and they sent a young girl out to help me. She was fortunate that there was a dishwasher but she still had a lot of work ahead of her. She cleaned the kitchen and cooked the dinner for us; supervised the children with their baths and pajamas. She came regularly for a while and was a great help. There were times when I was in such agony that I should have called an ambulance but the reason I did not was from fear that the family services department would take my children away from me; a prospect I simply could not face.

When I was able and strong enough to drive my children to school, I took extra painkillers and wore my sunglasses so they would not see the tears that my pain was causing me. To hold on to the wheel of the car was excruciating; the pain was unbearable and unbelievable. The stiffness reduced somewhat by midday, at least enough for me to get around a little more comfortably. The kitchen, however, had now become my enemy, and that included the Vegemite jar, as I could never manage to unscrew the lid. Such a simple task that any young child could easily master and yet for me, it was impossible. I stood alone many times at the kitchen sink in tears because my hands were too painful, stiff and weak to unscrew anything. I felt such hopelessness and aloneness having this disease that had turned me into a helpless cripple. I felt a level of despair at this point that I did not want to live in pain or sorrow anymore. If there had been access to a gun, I would have seriously considered using it. I was beyond the point of, "Who would love my children if I died?" The last thing I ever wanted, though, was for my children not to have a mother. I know all too well, what that feels like.

My mother abandoned me when I was an infant and I knew in the depths of my heart that I could not bear for my children to know what that feels like. My own tragic past was not going to deny my children a bright and successful future and the glory of life. I wanted them to know that nothing communicates more clearly than a mother's love. I wanted them to know and understand that I took pleasure in my presence being available to them at all times. It was what I lived for.

Meanwhile, my days—on the good ones—consisted of my children dressing me and taking me out to the kitchen for yet another day of painkillers, anti-inflammatory drugs, tears and anguish, and resting on the lounge in front of the television. My office chair was less cumbersome than a traditional wheel chair and sometimes my children would push me around the house on it, making a game for us, so that I could get from one room to another. I do not know how I would have survived without them. They prepared breakfast in the morning before school, and made the lunches with such enthusiasm while I watched over them. By late afternoon, there had been sufficient painkillers for me to manage the preparation of dinner. At that time, I also began making the school lunches so there was one less chore for them to do in the mornings.

Night time, however, was the worst. I managed about two to three hours sleep each night due to the pain, swelling, and stiffness in my shoulders, right knee, hands and wrists. The disease was also in my flesh and even the thought of a handbag over my shoulder was intolerable. To sleep at night was therefore impossible. It was all I could do to get through the night at all, let alone sleep. My children also knew not to lean up against my bed as it sent shockwaves through my entire being, leaving me wailing in pain. For me now, the most difficult thing of all was simply being alive.

Night time was also the loneliest time. I lay in the darkness of my room, alone with my thoughts, knowing I could not call out to my young ones, as God knows they needed their rest. Sometimes in the dark, I asked, "Oh lord have mercy on me" and in those tears I cried out, "Where is my miracle?" I lay motionless in my bed on my back not being able to move or roll over; reflecting back on my life and wondering if somehow emotional trauma could affect one's health. If there was one thing that I knew in the deepest recess of my heart, it was that emotional trauma affected one's spirit. In my bed alone with my thoughts, I thought that I would never recover from the way the disease had altered me, or shake off the despondency into which my personality had sunk. It seemed as if the hideous truth of the disease had paralyzed my spirit.

As the light of day dawned through the Venetian blinds, I dried my tears—hoping not to expose my sorrow in front of the children. They needed to feel safe in the strength that only a parent could offer. I wanted them to feel untouched by my illness. I wanted them to feel safe knowing I could still take care of them even if in a diminished capacity. I wanted them to know—mother—was still there for them, as frail as I was. My interest was merely to love them, to know them, to take care of them, to protect them. I believe I was born to love them, at least the best that I could with what I knew at the time. They were my life. Their love defined who I was. I did not want them to have any part in the burden of my sorrow.

Today was my children's sports day at school. They were so excited and looked forward to me being there. I told them if I could make it I would. But I knew it was impossible as I was just too sick and in too much pain. My son Ben could not contain his enthusiasm as sports were the main reason he looked forward to going to school. I did not want to disappoint him, but it was physically beyond me to get there. The sporting events started at nine and went till three and it was now eleven o' clock. I couldn't stop crying because of the pain and no amount of prescription drugs gave me any relief. Having an altruistic nature, I kept putting myself in my children's shoes and wanted to give them my presence on their special day. I thought, I may as well be in agony at the school, as home, so I took double the amount of pain killers, put on my sun glasses to hide my tears and off I went.

On my arrival at the school I noticed there were no parking spots left close by due to the amount of people attending the sports carnival, and the school gates were manned as we were not allowed to park on the school grounds. I knew I could not park a mile up the road as I was too sick and in too much pain to walk that distance back to the school entrance. I was desperate to get to my children as I knew how important it was to them that I attend. I decided to drive up to the school gates and tell them of my plight. It was obvious to them of my distress and they let me park in the school grounds close to the oval. I parked my car and carefully got out with tears streaming down my face. I opened up the boot of my car and took out my fold up chair for me to sit on. I turned around with my sun glasses still on hiding my red eyes from uncontrollable tears and saw that the oval was on higher ground than the school. This I had never noticed before.

I pondered on how I would climb this enormous hill, at least for me it was the highest hill in the world. It was my Everest. I stood alone as others went up and down around me. I struggled to step up on the rise, with my handbag over my painful flesh and the fold up chair in my right hand that screamed out in pain. I stood there and just wanted to die. I was so depressed and frustrated that my health had left me, and that I was reduced to being a helpless cripple living in such despair. In fact, I was grieving the loss of my health and my painful existence was becoming too much to bear.

People were buzzing all around me with the excitement of the day, the sun was shining and children were running and playing, screaming with enthusiasm as they participated in their sporting events, and yet for me, all I could do, was stand there. Suddenly, a little boy stopped upon noticing me, with his arm stretched out in front of him giving me a childish kind of wave and said, "Hello lady, my mummy's coming today." "You're a very lucky boy" I replied. It was then, and only then, I noticed that he was looking for her to see if she was still coming as it was already midday. I could see the hope in his eyes; I could see the unconditional love on his face for his mother. How this child and all children live for that love and approval from their parents, how the love of a parent defines who they are. For his sake, I hoped his mother came. I knew my attendance on this day was worth my effort, no matter how sick I was and how much easier it would have been for me to stay home in the face of my misery. This little boy reinforced for me how important I am to my children. How important my presence is on their special day. But, I didn't need the little boy to remind me how important a mother is to a child, having been raised in five different orphanages, children's homes and foster care for the first fourteen years of my life, I already knew.

Making a second attempt at climbing up onto the oval, I used my fold up chair as a support to get to my children. I walked along the oval struggling with my chair and handbag and with pain that would not go away. I couldn't stop the flow of tears because of my misery and especially the pain in my right knee. Then, my children spotted me and ran toward me with such happiness that I had arrived. The looks on their faces said it all. They helped me with my things and I sat in my fold up chair out of people's way, so I wouldn't be knocked in any way. I gave them money for their lunches, they were so excited. They brought me a cup of tea and a sandwich from the tuck shop. As they ran their events, they looked over at me for my approval, I waved and smiled and acknowledge them, letting them know how proud I was of them. It was truly a special time. For them, these memories are sweet and forever in their hearts.

As the months wore on, I got on with life the best I could. Sometimes that included doing the shopping at the mall. However, for most of the time, there was no shopping done. White as a sheet and drugged out of my mind with medication, without energy, trying to cope with the pain and, at the same time, hang on to a shopping trolley with hands that screamed in agony, it was literally all I could do to just remain upright. The fear of other shoppers accidentally knocking into me and touching my flesh as they passed was quite overwhelming. It was not until I was sick that I realized the aggressiveness of some shoppers. Their eyes and general demeanor spoke to me of their impatience, anger and aggression.

I did not have the strength to compete with them for space in the supermarket aisles. I was tired of my suffering and of the means by which I was forced to exist. I wanted to avoid others, to stay out of their way. My sunglasses hid the tears as I tried to round each aisle, only to give up in distress; a condition made worse by the knowledge that a task I once handled with ease had turned into such a huge chore.

I scrambled for the exit on many occasions, leaving my trolley where it stood and full of groceries, to escape being hurt or knocked; to look for a chair where I could rest my body. Sometimes kind strangers, upon noticing me, inquired how I was and asked if I would like a glass of water, or if they could call for an ambulance or a doctor. I always said yes to the water and no to the doctor and ambulance. Who would take care of my children with their mother in hospital? Because I spent my childhood in five different orphanages, I was terrified of my children being caught up in the welfare system as I was and never getting them back. Unfortunately, there were no relatives to call upon.

As sick and depressed as I was in grieving the loss of my health I could not, however, do what the doctors asked of me, to accept this disease and learn to live with it. My doctor offered me anti-depressants and sleeping tablets but, I refused the prescription as I felt I was drugged enough as it was. By this time I had reached such despair, I stayed away from doctors for almost twelve months, because I did not care to receive any more bad news and was quite ready to let this disease take me to my grave. In fact, I would have welcomed the relief. With the incessant pain, sleep deprivation, depression and chronic anemia, I did not care whether I lived or died.

Over time, the arthritis was taking hold and every part of my body and flesh screamed out in torment; indefinable pain and suffering was my constant companion. For a very long time my adorable children could not show me any physical affection, or touch me in any way unless invited to do so. I could only receive and give affection when I was sitting down on the lounge, prepared to receive a kiss on my cheek and to kiss them gently on theirs. They were not allowed to hug me as it was too painful to touch my flesh. What saddened me most of all was when night fell and it was time for bed, because I could not take my children by the hand and feel their flesh between my fingers as we headed for their bedroom; to wrap my arms around them; to hold them tight. To fill them up with a mother's physical love and affection; to sit on their beds and read them goodnight stories. To bend down at their bedside and kiss them goodnight, to stroke their faces and touch their hair, to give them butterfly kisses on their ears and their cheeks. The ritual had changed and it tugged at my heart for now I was the one they took to bed.

Before retiring, the children locked the house up at night and turned out the lights. By day, they went up to the corner shop for groceries on their bikes and still had time to tell me how sad they were I was sick, and how much they loved me. Their perpetual support, unconditional love and enthusiasm gave me the reason to go on. My love for them made me think about my life and the future that lay ahead. This disease had stolen the only mother they knew. Their love and support moved me deeply. Thoughts began to stir in my mind. I started to think about how I could become well. I reflected back on stories about people curing themselves of cancer through diet and nutrition. Could I not do the same for rheumatoid arthritis?

I knew deep down in my soul that I had to do something as time had exacerbated the illness and my ability to deal with it. The arthritis now affected my jaw, the back of my head, both shoulders, right elbow, both wrists, and hands—though not to the extent of deforming them. It affected both knees (there had been two operations on my right knee already and eventually my right arm was operated on, with the possibility of my left knee needing to be done in the future) and my weight loss was escalating along with muscle wastage. The disease had not left my eyes unscathed either; so inflamed were they by the arthritis that daylight caused them to weep and I could barely stand sunlight. In addition, sometimes in the middle of the night, I awoke to find it difficult to breathe. I was terrified of the arthritis getting into my lungs but I feel it was 'willed away' and the fear of this happening only occurred a few times over the years.

Looking in the mirror at my long 5'9"/175cm frame; gaunt through with muscle atrophy and rapid weight loss, which is part of the disease. I tried to re-assure myself but it was the self that others saw that was reflected back at me. I was always long and lean, so there was not much of a head start to begin with. Clearly, I could not afford to lose more weight. I became very self-conscious of my body as I felt everyone was judging me. I spent more and more time at home, and only went to the shops when it was unavoidable. My social life was nil and had been for years. My future was bleak and according to the doctors, rheumatoid arthritis was incurable and debilitating. They advised me that the sooner I accepted my illness and its prognosis, the better off I would be.

Their remarks saddened me, more for them than for myself. They have no hope or faith in the power of the human spirit or the power of the human mind when one is determined to succeed. Nor do they understand that given the right environment, a natural healing will take place within the body. If we are not born sick, surely it is the food we eat that makes us ill. Given the right nutrition, the body can reverse back to a healthy state. The immune system is more than capable of repairing and healing itself. This is what it is designed to do, if we let it. It was clearly obvious to me that taking the road of drug therapy meant that I would never recover, and only become worse loaded up on a cocktail of chemical toxins and then an early demise. I was already sick with a body in a very toxic state, why compound my problems by giving me more toxins?

Moreover, according to the doctors and the clinical evidence of RA, there was no future for me; I was in real trouble but something deep down inside of me would not, and could not, accept that I would end up like this for the rest of my life. The doctors call this denial. I call it hope. My determined attitude and tenacity caused me to never give up. To have believed the doctors meant that I would have to accept a life of misery, culminating in a premature death. For me this was unacceptable. I had too much to do, too many goals to achieve, my children's weddings to attend. Grandchildren to love and hold, and a personal goal I want to achieve—a dream I have had for years. Because of all this, I was not prepared to live in ill health and die long before my time. I had to introduce myself to new ideas on healing so I could turn my health around and enjoy not just good health, but excellent health.

Firstly, I had to find out everything I could on rheumatoid arthritis. Next, I read almost seventy books on diet and disease. Although, there was nothing out there to cure rheumatoid arthritis. Through trial and error plus a few set backs, I discovered the way to regain my lost health. It is this discovery; my journey that I wish to share with you. Fortunately, the memory of my pain has faded, for me it is over.

When I am out, I see the pain in your faces. I see the pain in your eyes, and I see the pain in your bodies. I recognize the symptoms, the disease. I could not live with myself or sleep at night with my new found health knowing there are too many of you who continue to be imprisoned by this disease. I wish for you to know my story so that you too can find your own courage to help yourself to freedom from rheumatoid arthritis. To help yourself to become who you were before this disease ravaged your body, to envision a future for yourself. To help yourself to become the person you were supposed to be. You can rise from the graveyard of your pain and live again—as you were meant to live; to give your life a purpose. When you do become well again, and I know you will, you will not be the person you were before. You will be stronger, wiser and more in tune with your body and your world. You will start to question what your purpose is, and why you are here in the first place. You do have a purpose; you are here for a reason. God does not make mistakes. You will have a greater appreciation of health, life, nature and animals. Life will be very different. It is giving yourself permission to believe you deserve it, and to believe it is possible for you.

After completing my research, it is horrific that doctors have no cure for rheumatoid arthritis. Not even their powerful drugs will eventually suppress the disease into oblivion. They simply mask the disease with chemicals that in the process can play havoc with your body. The side effects to the anti-rheumatic drugs are horrendous. I much preferred taking my chances with the disease based on a radical change of diet than to risk the side effects of drugs and their chemical components. From what I could see, patients who accept a doctor's prognosis, then go on a drug regime, one is only doomed to a life of misery and an early grave. But changing one's diet and mindset to accept and believe that the body can heal itself at least gives you a fighting chance. Imagine if you will, being well and pain free. Do not accept what is told to you about RA. It's thinking outside the square that sets you free.

The medical profession argues that the use of heavy rheumatic drugs for patients with rheumatoid arthritis early on in the disease will slow down and possibly prevent deformities before they occur. If this is true, then why do so many sufferers have deformities? Clearly, the drugs aren't working. "God" made our bodies with the intelligence to heal it self given the right stress free environment and nutrition? This is why we have an immune system. Only "God" can do this. Not drugs. Very little attention is being paid to what patients think. Some doctors are so caught up in their own expertise they fail to see what the patients want.

Emotional stress is a very big killer and the cause of many diseases. My childhood as I mentioned earlier was indeed extremely stressful and no doubt over those years of continued fear and violence toward me eventually took its toll.

The future belongs to those who believe
in the beauty of their dreams.
Eleanor Roosevelt

Things do not change; we change
Henry David Thoreau

Chapter 2

—*Testing Times*—

Emotional stress is one of the major contributing factors to my developing rheumatoid arthritis, not only because of my Western diet food, but because of the stressful life I had endured since infancy. Louise L Hay wrote in her book "Heal your Life" that arthritis is brought on by feeling unloved, criticism and resentment. I was unloved, criticized and felt resentment toward my perpetrators.

I spent the first fourteen years of my life in five different orphanages and children's homes, as well as foster care around Sydney, Australia from 1950 through 1964. The endless abuse and loneliness of those early years filled me with a perpetual melancholy and an indefinable loneliness that stretches back for as far as I can remember. Even now as a very mature woman, there remains a residual emptiness from those years that I do not know how to fill. As a result of my childhood being so brutal, I suffered from a condition known as traumatic amnesia for the first 41 years of my life. Not knowing any other way to digest the brutality meted out to me.

I have learnt as a mature woman from a psychotherapist that, once you reach the age of eighteen, you are totally responsible for your own life, and happiness. You can no longer blame your parents, for your childhood, or anything else that happened in your life for your problems now as an adult. We are in charge and it is up to us to get our lives in order. Easy said, you may think? Yes, it is easy said, but surely our upbringing sets us up, and prepares us for our future. Needless to say, if we keep blaming others for everything that happens in our lives, then that still gives them the power over our lives today. Furthermore, re-living our past and talking about it all the time, keeps us connected to the pain. If we take charge of our own lives and health, we take back our power and can forge ahead creating a positive future for ourselves. Therefore not remaining a victim, or having the victim mentality.

For me being on medication kept me a victim. After all, pumping chemical drugs into my body kept me a victim of the sickness industry. How on earth, can chemical poisons cure anything? It's absurd. Why should I have taken chemotherapy? I never had a methotrexate deficiency. I also never had a cortisone deficiency. Drugs suppress your immune system and take over. With out your immune system, you have nothing. You then become the victim of the drug companies.

I was a victim of my childhood, and I was a victim of rheumatoid arthritis and the sickness industry. Damned if I was going to remain one. The beauty of being healthy is you can do anything you want. When you lose the victim mentality you escape the clutches of your tormenters and perpetrators. You escape the clutches of your illness. You become empowered and then the sky is the limit. Think about a dream that you have always had, and then go for it.

I was told as a child that I was useless, ugly, and worthless and that I was possessed by the devil and was nothing more than a sinner. Imagine a six year old growing up with this kind of brainwashing, as well as the physical, mental, emotional and sexual abuse. Furthermore, there was medical neglect which almost cost me my life at the age of fourteen. By the time my twin sister walked me to the hospital from the orphanage, she was told I would have been dead with in the half hour. Is it any wonder I was suffering traumatic amnesia.

I was even deprived of a fantastic future playing tennis on the professional circuit and playing Wimbledon. The tennis coach that was hired to teach us at the last orphanage I was in, asked my mother if he could take me home to live with him and his family so he could coach me to Wimbledon, as he said he had never seen such a killer instinct in a player before. He said I hit the ball harder and more powerful than Yvonne Goolagong. My mother said, no. She didn't want me, but it was obvious she wasn't going to let anyone else have me either.

Although mother was never there for me as a child, except for the odd visit, I always loved her. I always craved her love. I craved for her to want me, to take me home with her. I just wanted her to acknowledge me, to own me. I tried to hate her, but I couldn't. A kind smile would have wiped away years of torment, and anguish. I would have forgiven her for anything. All she had to say was, "I love you." Sadly I was not to hear those words pass her lips. I never heard them. When she died at almost 82, reality set in, and I knew there was no hope of ever hearing those words. Strange as it may seem, once mother died, I thought the torment would be over. But it wasn't. A new kind of loneliness and sadness took over. Even though she was far from being protective and loving, once she was dead, I was crazy with grief and missed her terribly. She will be dead a very long time. Whilst she was alive, I had a mother, what ever that meant. All I could do was just get on with life, and live it the best way I could. One minute at a time, and one day at a time. I can't change what happened. She is long gone. What can I do? I can't keep blaming someone who is dead for all my problems, and there were many.

As a grown woman I have to be responsible for my own health, happiness, and my own future. Especially be responsible for what foods go into my mouth that can cause me to be sick. That is my responsibility. Not the doctors or anyone else.

God in his genius, as only he/she can do, designed us with a fabulous immune system to heal and repair the body. If you eat the right food, your immune system will take over, and heal your body. Just allow this to happen.

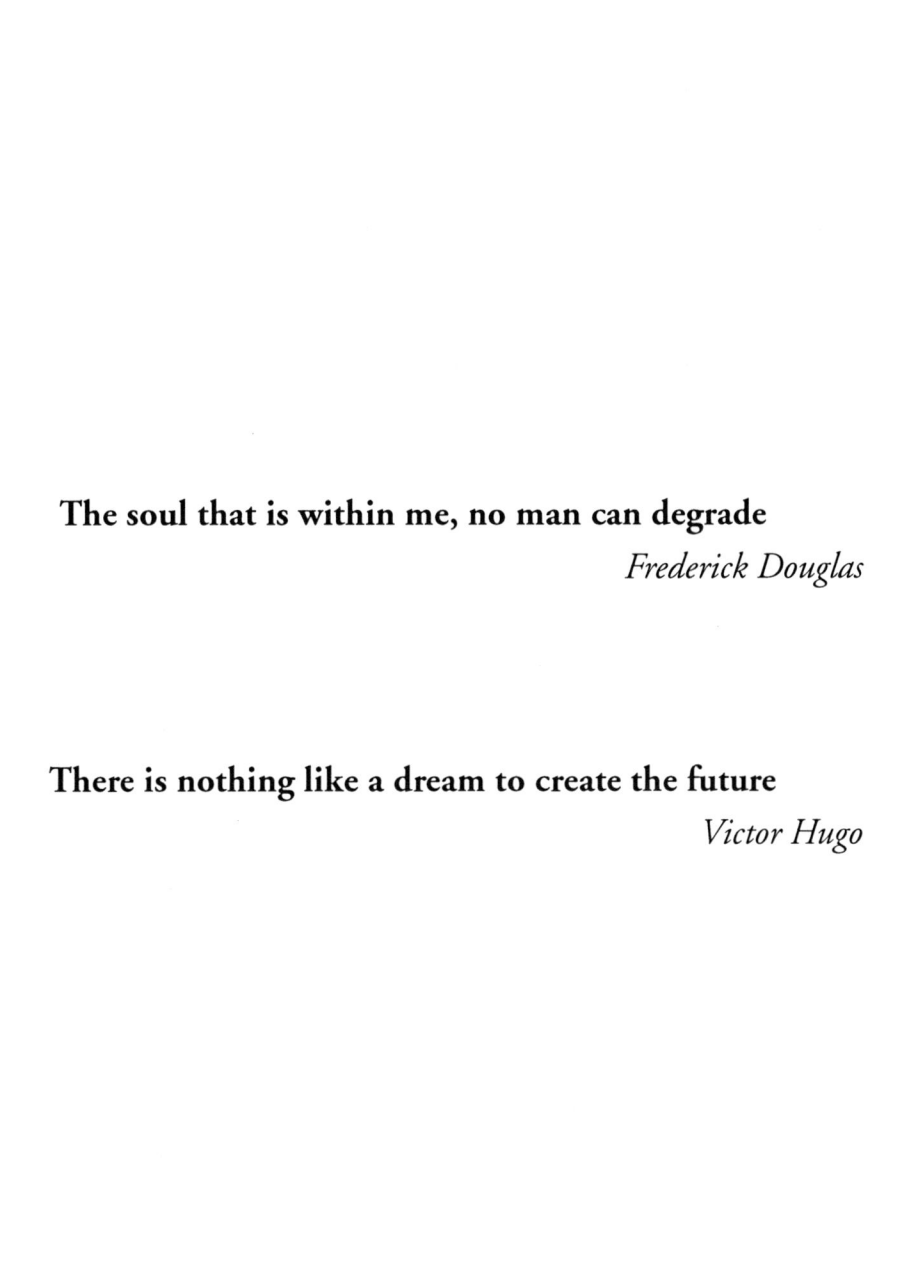

The soul that is within me, no man can degrade
Frederick Douglas

There is nothing like a dream to create the future
Victor Hugo

Chapter 3

—*Root Causes*—

By this time, you can well understand why I looked beyond powerful drug chemicals to the possibility of a more natural approach. I had already heard about many people curing themselves of cancer through diet high in fruit and vegetables, and maintaining a positive mental attitude. I began to read as many books as I could find on diet and disease. Many of the stories are extremely inspirational and motivating and some I have read several times.

According to the medical profession, treatment for RA entails the early intervention of anti-inflammatory and steroidal medication before the appearance of joint damage. However, we now know that diet plays a very important part in the prevention and cure of rheumatoid arthritis.

We have an example from as far away as half a century ago when the *Proceedings of the Royal Society of Medicine* (1936-1937) documented an experiment at the Royal Free Hospital in London using a restorative diet in the treatment of rheumatoid arthritis. In fact, reports from the Wayne State University Medical School document that when fat free diets were fed to six patients, all achieved a complete remission of the disease within seven weeks (Natural Health 1992.) Medical authorities say there are many different kinds of arthritis and the disease is so complex only highly trained specialists can treat it and even then, it is incurable.

This is utter nonsense. No matter the number of forms in which arthritis may present itself, there are only three major factors involved, two of them are dietary in origin and the third is stress. The dietary factors are blood fats and uric acid.

Arthritis has been suspected as being an autoimmune disease, one in which the white cells of the body actually attack the body 'by mistake'. White cells indeed are involved but like germs; they are blamed for mistakes made by the person who owns the body, who chooses to live on a high fat, high-protein diet (Horne 1988).

The white cells are of different types, the phagocytes being those that engulf foreign substances; germs etc., and destroy them with their powerful, corrosive, digestive juices. These white cells constantly patrol the tissues and joints of the body looking for any troublemakers.

Arthritis is caused in two ways. When, due to high fat levels in the blood and poor circulation, the oxygen level in the synovial fluid, which lubricates the joints, becomes so low that the white cells in that location perish, the cells disintegrate, and when they disintegrate, their corrosive digestive juices attack the joint and damage it. That is osteoarthritis. Gouty arthritis occurs the same way except that in this case the white cells are destroyed by crystals of uric acid, which precipitates in the blood primarily because of eating too much protein. Uric acid is normal in the blood in small quantities in solution but on a high protein diet, the concentration becomes so great that crystals precipitate, and these are needle-sharp so when ingested by the white cells, the cells are punctured and destroyed. High blood fat levels exacerbate the uric acid problem by virtue of the fact they impede the clearance of the acid from the bloodstream.

The two processes, of course, may occur simultaneously and will be exacerbated by stress that causes an increase in blood fats and blood viscosity. Bread, alcohol and refined sugar are other exacerbating factors. The calcium build-up that occurs at the joints is due to the body's efforts of self-protection when calcium is taken from the bones to counteract the high acid levels. Herein, of course, lays the cause of osteoporosis, the disease in which the bones become de-calcified.

The same destructive processes that result in arthritis cause rheumatism when tissues other than the joints are affected. However, remember that emotional stress also plays a very important part in inducing arthritis.

As in so many other diseases, emotional stress is often a major factor in rheumatoid arthritis through its disruptive effect on the hormonal system and its effect of elevating blood fats. In his book *Mind and Body* (William Kimber, London, 1969), Dr. Stephen Black states that the incidence of this disease is seven times greater among women than among men. He described how, in the majority of cases, women are the intelligent active personality type who frustrated by the role in life in which they find themselves, and unhappy in their relationships with men (Horne 1983).

Stress can induce arthritis because adrenaline causes a rapid rise in free fatty acids in the blood. Refined carbohydrates, deficient in vitamins, produce the same effect on the body as stress and when consumed as part of a diet, are often responsible for triggering an attack of arthritis. White bread is bad, even wholegrain bread, and other acid forming cereal foods are just as conducive to arthritis.

Dr. Loris Chahl of Queensland University is investigating the relationship between mental stress and various inflammatory ailments, such as skin rashes and arthritis. She said her research was "getting somewhere" and that if a connection was proved, it would help to explain many clinical problems, to quote again from Dr. Dintenfas (Horne 1988).

Medical treatment for arthritis is useless. In gouty arthritis, gold salts are sometimes injected as treatment. The white cells that envelop the gold particles instead of uric acid crystals, cannot digest them either and so are immobilized, but do not burst. In some cases there may be some relief experienced by the patient.

Cortisone will destroy white blood cells and perhaps relieve some symptoms but is otherwise harmful. The body has an essential need for white cells. They are vital. Aspirin may relieve arthritis too, by its effect on suppressing the white blood cells; X-rays can also kill white cells. With inactive white cells, colds and infections will persist.

On the other hand, as with other metabolic diseases, the adoption of correct diet reverses arthritis. A very low saturated fat, low protein diet that contains lots of fresh fruits and fresh vegetables is the answer, preferably eaten raw. Acid forming cereals and legumes, as well as meat, eggs and dairy products should be avoided (Horne 1988). All animal protein foods tend to be harmful in a number of ways.

Meat and animal by-products, i.e. dairy foods, introduce too much protein into the diet, and they contain too much fat and cholesterol. When cooked they produce cancer inducing chemicals and are devoid of enzymes. They are also devoid of fiber and therefore cause constipation.

The fat content of meat increases enormously when beef cattle are raised in stalls and fattened with the use of hormones and overfeeding. However, long before meat producers adopted this practice observant medical men had noted the marked, adverse effects of eating meat.

Dr. Arnold Lorand of Austria in his book, *Old Age Deferred* (1910) devoted an entire chapter to the "Dangers of an Abundant Meat Diet." He observed, and quoted a number of other medical researchers who corroborated his findings (Horne 1988.)

Although Dr. Arnold Lorand devoted an entire chapter to the adverse effects of eating meat back in 1910, I came across a book in my research that devotes the entire book to the adverse effects of eating meat and dairy products, which are animal by-products. The book is titled *Mad Cowboy—Plain Truth from the Cattle Rancher who Won't Eat Meat*, and is written by Howard F. Lyman with Glen Merzer, published in 1998.

Howard F. Lyman, reared on a dairy farm and cattle ranch in Montana, USA, states that if you are a meat-eater in America, you have a right to know that you have something in common with most of the cows you have eaten: they have eaten meat, too.

Moreover, according to Heart surgeon Dr. Mehmet C, Oz, (author of 'You' The owners manual) who assisted in the heart by-pass surgery of Bill Clinton, he states that meat actually rots in your gut. Therefore, high protein and saturated fat diets cause high blood pressure which causes kidney damage and impotence. In fact, my own rheumatologist told me years ago that meat inflames the body. This is why it is so important to eat anti-inflammatory foods and meat is not one of them.

Let food be your medicine and medicine be your food
Hippocrates

Watermelon—it's a good fruit. You eat, you drink, and you wash your face.
Enrico Caruso

Chapter 4

—*Where death begins*—

From all the books I read on diet and disease, I realized that death starts in the colon and a good way of cleansing your colon was to drink watermelon juice.

For example, for three months over one summer I drank only fresh watermelon juice every morning, (about three to four glasses) until midday when I ate lunch. Within three weeks my colon was cleansing itself naturally with loose motions (which is a sign of detoxification) four to five times a day and watermelon is a lot cheaper than having colonics. By the third week, I started passing black, shiny, tar-like motions several times a day and the evacuations were powerful. This lasted another three weeks before the color went back to normal.

I was not frightened by what was happening to me, as I instinctively knew it was all a part of the detoxification process. However, I was not sure what the black, shiny tar-like motions indicated although I knew, intuitively, it was nothing sinister. One day I was browsing through a bookstore, a favorite pastime, when I picked up a book called, *Tissue Cleansing Through Bowel Management* by Dr. Bernard Jensen, D.C., Ph.D., Nutritionist.

As I was looking through his book, I could not believe what I saw. There were colored pictures of people's stools long like rope that were black, and shiny like tar. The same that I had passed for a period of three weeks, four to five times a day was in fact, residue from childhood that had adhered to the colon wall as plaque does to blocked arteries. I was amazed at the results. I cleansed myself at such a deep cellular level, I passed years and years of deposits on just watermelon juice without even realizing the positive effects it would have on me. More importantly, the positive effect it would have on my health.

Mother Nature can detoxify your body naturally for very little money. I do believe, however, in enemas when you are on a juice or water fast only, especially for cancer patients. If you have a doctor or nurse in the family or you are not adverse to giving yourself enemas then, by all means, have at least one enema a day, preferably two; one in the morning, and one at night. What is important is that when you are detoxifying you need at least one bowel motion a day to clear out the toxins that have been brought down from deep cellular level into the bloodstream for elimination. Otherwise, you may suffer severe detoxification symptoms. Do not buy chemical laxatives, as they can be dangerous to your health.

In other words, Mother Nature will take care of everything naturally, given the right environment. Incidentally, my aim is to help people to help themselves the natural way without spending thousands of dollars to get well. You will regain your health if you move back to Mother Nature and eat plenty of fruit and vegetables; organic if you can afford them—but be careful as some health food stores sell commercial food as organic. One health food store, in particular, on the Gold Coast in Queensland has been cited on three occasions for selling commercially grown produce as organic. I restored my health by eating commercial produce as organic food was out of my price range and I do not have a green thumb, (everything I touch in the garden turns brown). It's best to source out your local organic markets and buy fresh organic produce from the growers. I now eat only organic fresh food. It is superior to commercial food sprayed with chemicals and pesticides.

As I was not sure of what I was doing in the early days and had no confidence in my own ability to get well, I turned to other methods. For example, I went to a health retreat in a rural part of Sydney. They put me on a fast for seven days that permitted only water. By the third day, I could hardly get out of bed and had lost interest in drinking any water at all. I managed to drink two to three glasses a day as otherwise I knew I could die from my own toxins. I was in a severe state of detoxification, no doubt due to the chemical drugs I took for the arthritis. I asked why they would not give me any enemas to clear out the toxins so I would not feel so ill and they said it was not necessary as when it was all over I would eventually 'go' without that assistance.

By the fifth day, I begged to be given food as I could barely lift my head up off the pillow. They talked me into continuing for the whole seven days, as this would be very beneficial. I was too weak to argue. I knew I was in a serious state of detoxification and felt like I was dying. I was very disappointed and upset that they would not listen to me and give me enemas, which are of paramount importance when you are on a water or juice only fast for that length of time. Once the toxins have been removed at deep cellular level and have entered the bloodstream for elimination, it is imperative that you have a daily bowel motion; otherwise, you can end up in serious trouble.

Between day five and day seven of my water only fast, I could not even lift my head off the pillow and was as weak as a kitten. What scared me the most was that I had lost all control and did not even desire to drink any water at all. I am only sorry that I could not ring an ambulance and be taken to hospital where I would have at least been given a drip to hydrate my body. Moreover, I lost an enormous amount of weight and as I was already underweight because one of the symptoms of RA includes rapid weight loss, I looked like death.

On day seven, I demanded food immediately as I was now frightened by my condition. Over the next seven days I regained enough strength to fly back home to the Gold Coast in a wheel chair. They insisted I stay another week to recover more strength, and they were right, I was really in no condition to go anywhere, but I just wanted to get the hell out of there. My children and friends could not believe my condition. I looked anorexic. I did not leave the house for months until I had gained enough weight to look almost normal though still very thin. As we live close to a shopping centre, my children did the shopping for me by pushing the trolley home every week. I do not know what I would have done without them.

In my opinion the health retreat's biggest mistake was not giving me enemas when putting me on strict water fasts. What they did to me was downright dangerous and life threatening. Dr. Paavo Airola states that this is the reason that virtually all biological doctors in Europe administers enemas to all fasting patients—once, twice and even three times a day. He goes onto say that, during fasting, enemas will assist the body in its cleansing and detoxifying effort by washing out all the toxic wastes from the alimentary canal (Airola 1971). In fact, Dr. Airola has seen rather horrifying examples of what prolonged water fasting without enemas can do. He treated a patient once who had been in a famous American clinic where he fasted for 32 days on water only. During all this time, he was advised to stay in bed, with the exception of short periods of sunbathing. He was given no enemas or colonic irrigations and it took him two months to 'recuperate' from this fast and get on his feet. He was still in a very weak condition with damaged kidneys and severe edema in his legs (Airola 1971).

In some fasting clinics around the world, enemas are given morning and night. Alternatively, juices are given one day and raw food the next day that, in turn, stimulates the peristalsis of the bowel by the eating of the food. Therefore, a natural bowel movement takes place. I could not agree more as I believe things are meant to happen naturally. Sometimes nature needs a little help, especially when fasting only on juices or water for several days. However, it is for the short term only. This is why my mission in life is to help people to help themselves *naturally* for the least amount of money.

People accept that the stiffness and pain of arthritic joints are an inevitable part of growing old but is arthritis part of normal aging? A cleansing regime based on fresh uncooked foods gives the body a chance to dispel the misery-causing toxins responsible for painful joints. The only way to do this naturally is to eat lots of raw foods, including fresh fruits, salads, nuts, seeds and fresh vegetables.

The idea is to get back to nature. We have allowed ourselves to become so far removed from nature that we are all becoming ill. Our Western food habits and dietary regimes will only kill you in the long run, and more likely in the short run. You may ask why some people eat as they please and live to be very old. It all boils down to the body's ability to eliminate toxic waste effectively. I knew of a man who, every time he ate a meal, (three times a day) went afterwards straight to the toilet for a bowel movement. He was like a baby, in one end and out the other. Constipation is what is killing us and Western diet food is very constipating.

High saturated fats, sugar, grains, table salt, preservatives, colorings and flavorings are not conducive to good health. White foods such as white flour, sugar and white rice are included in the problem. The *New Scientist* has reported on trials in China where one in ten adults die from liver cancer caused by aflatoxin, a toxin produced by moulds growing in rice and cereal grains. (New Idea August 11, 2001.) The food industry has a lot to answer for but, unfortunately, everything is about money.

Another substance detrimental to our health is prescription medication, which is authorized far too freely by some doctors. Confirmation of this fact was aired on the 7am news, Radio 92.5 Gold F.M, Gold Coast, July 18, 2002 to the effect that 140,000 people a year have a significantly adverse reaction to prescription medications as to require hospitalization in Australia alone.

What amused me was the inference that it was the fault of those who experienced such reactions that millions of taxpayer dollars are expended in remedying these problems. What should have been said was that it is the attitude of international pharmaceutical monoliths, in conjunction with a largely compliant medical fraternity, who are responsible for this problem with prescription medication. People need to understand that chemical drugs cause harm to the human body that eventually result in adverse reactions. When it comes to managing our own bodies and our own health, the belief that everyone else is right, and that chemical prescriptions are a normal part of our life, is programmed into our way of looking at things. I prefer to reclaim control over my body and my health. It is much safer in my hands.

If I listened to the doctors and kept taking drugs I would have probably been on the medication Vioxx, which has now been recalled world wide because doctors have now discovered it doubles your risk of heart attack and stroke, especially after eighteen months of use. There were three million prescriptions for Vioxx written each year for arthritis sufferers. My gut instinct told me years ago to fear the chemical drugs rather than my disease.

In addition, according to the journal of American medical association in a recent study, tens of millions of people are injured by prescription drugs, and just fewer than 1 million people die every year by these dangerous poisons in the United States. Moreover, Dr. Julian Whitaker, states that millions of us swallow pills that are supposed to make us feel better—physically or mentally—but covertly wreak havoc with our body and brain and many older folks are dismissed as senile, when in fact, their drugs are causing their memory lapses and confusion. What we call side effects of legal drugs are in fact diseases brought on by the medication.

Also, Nobel prize winning chemist, Linus Pauling, predicted that the use of toxic chemicals to suppress disease symptoms, which he called a toximolecular approach, was a blind alley that would lead nowhere, where it has lead, is to a catastrophically expensive and ineffective disease-care system, where people are killed and injured daily, where they remain chronically ill and where the costs are projected to double in the next ten years.

Dr. Joseph Mercola author of the book "Total Health" states, and I quote with his permission, *"though drugs are sometimes appropriate and at times can save a person's life, most of the time they are unnecessary, harmful and expensive.*

In my opinion, drug companies are driven by profits and have used their power to influence many areas of medicine. What is most unfortunate is that this has resulted in many biased studies, which ultimately lead to misleading information to the public.

The drug companies' intentions are evident in the $3 billion that was spent in 2002 for advertising costs and the vast amounts of money they donate toward grants and scholarships used to fund the costs of medical schools. Their motives don't stop there as they are also spending about $15 billion a year on physician marketing.

And while doctors play a role in the drugging of America, it's not completely their fault. Most physicians have no clue that the drug companies are spending (on average) $10.000 per doctor to influence their behavior. The doctors, of course, do not receive a check, but the perks can be quite significant.

One of the books in this article touches on all these aspects: "The truth about Drug Companies: How they Deceive us and What to Do About it," by Dr. Marcia Angell. Dr. Mercola also goes on to say that he recommends the book "Trust Us We're Experts."

Related Articles:

Drug firms Ignore Federal Law, Not Reporting Studies

How Could Drug Companies be so Evil?

U.S. Drug Researcher Imprisoned for FDA Fraud

Odds Are The Drug Industry is Paying Off Your Doctor

Questions Arise on U.S. Drug Policy" (end of quote.)

What lies behind us and what lies before us are tiny matters compared to what lies within us
Ralph Waldo Emerson

Some cause happiness wherever they go; others whenever they go.
Oscar Wilde

Chapter 5

—*Natural Solutions*—

From the time I told my rheumatologist I was going to cure myself of RA and that I had changed my diet to one that did not include meat, he asked me where I would get my iron from. I replied, "From the same place cows get theirs, plant food." We all know what happens when cows eat meat or flesh as was discussed earlier in this book. They get mad cow disease. (Perhaps mad cow is the animal version of Alzheimer's and schizophrenia?)

In fact, in 2003, the 9am News on Radio 92.5 Gold FM, Queensland carried an item on February 18, that scientists have now discovered some 70% of meat and dairy eaters are at high risk of developing Alzheimer's disease and that people should eat a diet high in vegetables and nuts. This was not news to me as according to my research some doctors and natural therapists have known this for years, even as far back as the early 1900s. There is now every good reason to think seriously about changing your eating habits to a more natural regime, especially if you want to regain your lost health. The only nuts I eat are chemical free almonds, walnuts, Brazil nuts, macadamia, and raw unsalted cashews. Also, on October 18, 2002 scientists discovered that backyard chooks pecking at pesticides and fertilizer produce toxins in their eggs causing ovarian cancer. Another reason to eat plant food.

The European tradition of using uncooked foods to heal and to promote high-level health continues to thrive at such famous clinics as the Bircher-Benner (Zurich), Ringberg (Tergensee, West Germany) and Biologisches Sanatorium

In other words, the universal cure for just about any ailment is the eating of 'living foods.' Raw food cured the German physician Max Gerson, a near contemporary of Bircher-Benner, of his migraine headaches. He thought if his monkey ancestors had lived healthily on fruit, nuts and green vegetables, so could he. Max Gerson was considered one of the most eminent and exceptional intellectuals in medical history.

Max Gerson went on to treat all his patients with uncooked food, including patients suffering from lupus and cancer. He became most famous for his book *A Cancer Therapy: Results of Fifty Cases* first published in 1958.

One of my favorite books on healing through nature is Ross Horne's *'Improving on Pritikin.'* It states that over a hundred years ago Dr Emmet Densmore and his wife, who was also a medical doctor, collaborated to write a book called *How Nature Cures*. In this book, the fallacies surrounding orthodox medicine were exposed and in support of his opinions, Dr Densmore quoted some of the prominent physicians of the time who, like the Densmores, had awakened to the fact that orthodox medicine for the treatment of common diseases was a waste of effort that frequently bordered on the farcical.

Dr Robert Mendelsohn writes that children have a natural fearful instinct regarding doctors and medication. It reminded me of my fear of the rheumatic drugs that were being offered to me. I was more afraid of the drugs than the disease. I instinctively knew the medication would do me more harm than good. I was not afraid of the disease, whereas I guess most people do have fear. I would rather the disease take me than the side effects of the drugs. At least with the arthritis, I knew what I was dealing with; with the drugs I did not.

Not only was I not afraid of the disease, I knew all along I would recover, somehow, someway. I believed in me. I did not blindly believe in the doctors, nor do I blindly believe in anyone. Because of my childhood, I soon discovered not to trust anyone. I have faith in me, my natural instincts and my intuition that I always listen to and act upon. When I first told my rheumatologist that I would cure myself of this disease he looked at me and said nothing. He did not say that this disease is incurable, but I knew he believed it. Even on my worst days when I visited him for pain killing injections into my joints. I always told him that I would cure myself through diet and that I would recover. He said to me "If nothing else Sonia, you have a very positive attitude and that is the main thing." I know he never believed me in the beginning. But as time wore on he could not believe how my health was not deteriorating. He once told me—I was amazing, (meaning, what I was doing for my health.)

I took that as a compliment and I think he started to come around and began to believe in what I was doing. Of course, I do not know of this for certain, as it must be a difficult proposition for doctors to admit their patients can turn their own health around, let alone a supposedly incurable crippling auto-immune disease like rheumatoid arthritis. Sometimes he asked me what I was eating. In fact, on one visit when I was feeling well I said to him again, "You know Doctor, I will beat this disease." He replied, "You already have." In order for me to survive, I needed to be in control of my own health, my own body, and my own life. I have more faith in me and my determination and strength to take care of me because I know—faith *can* move mountains. I believed in me when no one else did.

▶ HORMONE REPLACEMENT THERAPY

When I was first diagnosed as peri-menopausal, my symptoms were severe. I had extreme lethargy and no interest in life or domestic duties. I had a headache that felt like the top of my head was going to explode at any given moment. I was depressed and even suicidal. Unlike some women where their levels drop subtly over a period of years creating little or no symptoms, my doctor reported that my hormone levels had taken a nose dive. He offered me HRT and I refused, telling him I would prefer to do it naturally. He said to me, "You'll be back." I said, "no I won't." Within a month, I was back for HRT, as I was not coping at all. In fact, I had become worse. I was so vague I could not find a street address without difficulty. I could not believe what was happening to me. The thought of putting one foot in front of the other to get to the letter box was exhausting. I was only 40 years old and felt like an old woman. In those days, I, like most people, thought chemical drugs was the answer to everything.

Within three days on HRT, I was back to normal. I asked the doctor how women coped in the old days with such severe menopausal symptoms. He said, "They locked them up and threw away the key, and with your symptoms you would have been one of them."

With the diagnosis of rheumatoid arthritis a few years later, I did not notice at first the effect that HRT had on my pain. However, after my body had detoxified over a few years, my blood tests had improved dramatically and my pain was negligible, the effects of HRT became pronounced. Every time I took Provera or Primilut (a chemical progesterone) for the first ten days of the month on HRT I ended up in severe pain, especially in my wrists and shoulders. My daughter had to start dressing me again because I could not lift my arms up away from my side. At first, I thought it was RA returning due to something I had eaten. I blamed tomatoes and gave them up, even though I had been eating them all along.

Then I realized that within two to three days on Primilut there was a lot of pain and by the tenth day it was much worse. Within a few days to a week after coming off Primilut the pain disappeared. I took notice from then on and every month the same thing happened. Eventually, I discovered that HRT—which included the chemical drug Primilut (chemical progesterone) made the inflammation worse, in fact, it brought on joint pain. I decided not to take Primilut every month, but stretch it out to every six to ten weeks to avoid the pain though I knew my increased risks of cervical cancer on HRT. I came off the Estrogen patch slowly by using the patch three days on and then three days off for many weeks.

After eleven years, due to the pain of the arthritis and associated health risks, I decided to come off HRT. I had tried a couple of times before to come off 'cold turkey' and had ended up with a recurrence of the previous severe symptoms. This time I went to my new doctor, who practices nutritional medicine, and asked her what else could be done to help alleviate my symptoms. She suggested I use a natural progesterone cream as opposed to the chemical progesterone primulit, or provera to help ease the hot flushes. Within two days of using the cream, I was in agony and could not raise my arms again due to the pain in my shoulders. Again, my daughter had to dress and undress me for a few days until I cut back on the amount of cream I used but I still had pain. I decided to stop the cream altogether and the pain went. There is a natural HRT which I tried, and within six weeks I felt normal for the first time in a long time and without any hot flushes. Unfortunately, even the natural progesterone gives me joint pain.

Freedom is what this book is about: freedom from chemical drugs, freedom from rheumatoid arthritis and freedom from ill health; freedom to be able to do as we please which we cannot do if we are crippled with RA. Freedom to continue to work; to achieve our goals, to move without pain. Freedom to define ourselves in any way we wish; freedom to be able to climb the ladder of success, to achieve our goals and our dreams. Freedom to become the person you were meant to be.

The greatest thing a man can do in this world is to make the most possible out of the stuff that has been given him. This is success, and there is no other.
Orison Swett Marden

The destiny of man is in his own soul
Herodotus

Chapter 6

—*Recovery in Context*—

Assiduous adherence to the recovery diet is essential if you want to become well. There is no easy way around it, nor are there any quick fixes. It has taken us years to develop the level of toxins in our individual bodies that are now making us ill and it will therefore take time for reversal and healing to occur. However, given the right environment a natural remission can take place.

All packaged and canned food has to go because we need to get back to basics. We are so far removed from Mother Nature it is no wonder that we are developing 'civilized' diseases, disorders and syndromes. Even our domesticated pets suffer from our diseases because of what we feed them. Animals in the wild, living on their natural foods, are very lean with no weight problems and do not develop human illnesses. In fact, their immune system is stronger in the wild.

You need to stay on the recovery regime until you are free of pain and this natural healing can take at least twelve months. Everybody is different and we all detoxify at a different rate and depending on what medication you are taking. Some medications interfere with the detoxification process, especially blood pressure tablets and chemical or natural progesterone. For this reason, it is imperative that you find yourself a doctor who practices nutritional medicine so that you can gradually be taken off your medication as you become well. Do not attempt, to come off your medication abruptly, particularly cortisone, because you can develop adrenal shut down that can cause death.

After a period on the recovery diet, you will not need blood pressure tablets as your blood pressure will start to normalize as your body is slowly detoxifying and clearing out your toxins that caused you to become unwell.

Do not continue to see a doctor who does not believe in what you are doing and who will not help you come off your medication. Many doctors believe in detoxifying the body. Search them out for they are out there. Because many patients are seeking alternative therapies, a number of doctors are now practicing naturopaths as well as general physicians. Most doctors, however, are trained skeptics and you therefore need to be aware that it is your responsibility to be aware of, and to take control of your own body and health. Be the master of your own health and destiny; dare to reach for all that you imagine.

Next time you visit a doctor, ask for a copy of all your blood tests, including updates. Keep an eye on your reports and watch the improvements over time. This will excite you and help keep you motivated as the pain decreases. It will also give you the incentive to keep going and empower you to take back the control over your own life. If it's your belief that your doctor is taking care of you and that is how you like it, ask yourself the question, "How is it working for me?"

Once you start to feel a little better do not make the mistake of having just a little of your old favorite foods. You will undo some of the good you have already done and the pain will return.

Once your blood tests are completely normal and you are in a full remission, you can start introducing other foods to your diet and then follow the maintenance regime. If you resume your old eating habits, you will pay the price. You cannot risk taking any chances, not if you wish to enjoy excellent health and longevity.

An elderly man I knew who was in his seventies and suffered from rheumatoid arthritis was telling me a story about his older brother who also had the disease while in his early seventies who went on a diet many years earlier. Apparently, his brother had found a diet regime in an old book from the library and recovered from RA after only twelve months. The brother was so excited about his new found health and energy, which he had not enjoyed since his twenties, that he decided to 'go bush' and take up pig shooting.

He not only shot the wild boar—he ate it. He ate every kind of food he thought he had been missing. He thought his newly found health could never again be compromised because he felt so energetic, alive and well. His arthritis did not come back, but six years later, he died of cancer of the pancreas. The message is that we must not take our bodies and our health for granted, especially when we are given a second chance. Remember, if we find one small excuse for ourselves to go off our diet, we will soon find a hundred more and will quickly revert to just what we were before.

I now look upon my body as a God given temple to house my spirit and I surely intend to look after it. I walk on my treadmill every day for a minimum of 30 minutes. I mix with positive, motivated people. You need to believe in yourself and not allow well meaning friends, relatives and loved ones to negate your own innate wisdom. Start to believe in yourself and become a positive thinker. Stay away from dream killers, and surround yourself with a dream team. Your continued positive attitude and awareness of your own internal dialogue will dictate how well you will become.

You will not believe how forgiving the body is and how it will repair itself and take you again to a healthy state, once you commence eating a high raw food diet, years are added to your life. You will not believe your increased energy. Men can even reverse impotency once the artery to the penis is unblocked through a highly nutritious diet. Once you give up smoking, alcohol and the typical Western diet you will be able to smell and taste your food once again. You will become sensitive to the smells of your environment and add quality years to your life. Never allow yourself the luxury of a negative thought. Moreover, be aware of self sabotage as you start to feel better, because your old thinking patterns will continue to re-surface unless you are devoted to getting yourself well.

In fact, ask for spousal and family support, as it will go a long way in helping you to recover. Perhaps they could join you on the diet and be amazed at the benefits to their own health and well-being. Try to break the habit of taking medication every time you get a cold, flu, headache or sore throat. Your body will take care of you provided you give it plenty of water and nutrition. For instance, some headaches are caused simply by the lack of water (which can also be a sign of dehydration). Whatever the nature of your health problem, you will feel fantastic once you start on a highly nutritious high raw food regime—and stick to it!

▶ ARTHRITIS

According to the Australian arthritis foundation 3.4 million Australians suffer arthritis at the cost of $11.2 billion dollars to the tax payer each year. The American arthritis foundation states some 70 million Americans suffer one form or another of arthritis and 2.1 million Americans specifically suffer from rheumatoid arthritis. In addition, in America there are 300,000 children with some form of arthritis. The following is a list of the types of arthritis that plague our modern day society:

    Anklylosing Spondylitis
    Arthropathy
    Ehler's-Canlos Syndrome
    Enthesopathy
    Fibromyalgia
    Juvenile Ankylosing
    Juvenile Dermatomysoitis
    Juvenile Enteropathic Arthritis
    Juvenile Non-Inflammatory disorders
    Juvenile Psoriatic Arthritis
    Juvenile Reactive Arthritis
    Juvenile Reiter's Syndrome
    Juvenile rheumatoid Arthritis (JRA)
    Soft tissue Hydated Disease
    Spondylitis
    Systemic Lupus Erythematosus (SLE)
    Vascular Necrosis

Juvenile Scleroderma
Juvenile Spondyloarthopathy
Juvenile Systemic Lupus Erythematosus
Juvenile Vasculitis
Lyme Disease
Marfan Syndrome
Osteoarthritis
Osteoporosis
Pauciarticular JRA
Polyarticular JRA
Psoriatic Arthritis
Raynaud's Phenomenon
Rheumatoid Arthritis (RA)
Sarcoidosis
Scleroderma
Sea Juvenile Syndrome
Seronegativity

These are just some of the many forms in which arthritis manifests, most of them auto-immune based. The really frightening and depressing thing about autoimmune diseases is that although one could initially be diagnosed with rheumatoid arthritis, it could then mutate into Systemic Lupus Erythematosus (SLE) or Scleroderma.

This information, plus the constant injunction from doctors, "to go home and learn to live with it" made me very frustrated. What I needed most from the doctors was their help in actually recovering from the disease. It was never forthcoming.

▶ DIABETES

Some RA sufferers suffer multiple health problems including high blood pressure, angina, heart disease and diabetes. It is *imperative* that you consult a doctor who practices nutritional medicine to help you come off your medication gradually, or at least to determine a minimal dosage. If you stay with a doctor who does not support your new attitude to food then your medication could interfere with you becoming completely well. Try and find yourself another doctor who will help you with this diet. In fact, a Swedish research team discovered that half a teaspoon of cinnamon per day will lower blood sugar levels naturally for type 2 diabetes—researchers have found that cinnamon contains a bioactive component with "insulin-like" effects. Fresh cinnamon would be the best. This diet will enable you not to need any medication at all.

▶ STROKES

If you have suffered a stroke and you are on Warfarin blood thinning medication, you will need to speak to your doctor before you start this diet. The diet itself will not cause you harm, as I have never known anyone to die from eating fruit and vegetables. It is the interference of the chemical drug Warferon with the natural vitamin K in the healthy food you need to consume that could cause you harm. I know a lady who was visiting her husband in hospital, when a man in the next bed said to her that he was on a chemical blood thinning medication similar to Warfarin, that caused him to have a nose bleed that would not stop, he was admitted to hospital for several days in order for the bleeding to be controlled. Chemical drugs can be down right dangerous and simply unnecessary

If you really want to become healthy and rid yourself of rheumatoid arthritis and its insidious deformities and chronic unrelenting pain, it is paramount that you seek a doctor who practices nutritional medicine, in order for you to gain the benefits from this diet. The mother of a friend of mine came off Warferon successfully so that she could lead a healthier life. Vitamin E is a natural blood thinner but also, should be used with caution.

If you follow this diet strictly, and stay off Western diet food, your blood pressure will naturally drop to a more normal level and you will not need anticoagulants to thin your blood. Nor, will you need high blood pressure medication. You will be surprised at the health benefits you will gain. You can say goodbye to constipation, heartburn, high blood pressure, obesity, type 2 diabetes, lupus and rheumatoid arthritis.

▶ STIFF AND PAINFUL JAW

If you can hardly eat any food due to the pain and stiffness in your jaw, try a little pureed vegetables, mashed banana, grated apple, and any other fruit you can tolerate (except for high acid fruits) that does not require much mastication. Also, drink fruit juices, pure water and herbal tea until you are in less pain and can tolerate the chewing of other food on the menu. If you can, try some organic dried fruit such as apricots, raisins and sultanas. (Soak them in purified water for a couple of hours to soften for easier mastication) Do not eat dried fruit that is not organic because they usually contain vegetable oil and sulphur. Do not eat orange colored dried apricots. Organic dried apricots are black. As of 2004 vegetable oil has been discovered to cause macular degeneration (blindness) and cancer. Recently I met an elderly woman at a talk I gave, who in fact, been told by her eye specialist that she developed macular degeneration from eating vegetable oil. Not to educate people about this product is down right neglect. To know about it, is one thing. But to meet someone in the flesh who is blind because of this oil is criminal. I have not eaten vegetable oil since I first changed my diet back in 1996. The only oils I will eat are; organic coconut oil, cold pressed extra virgin olive oil, and apricot oil. Only use organic coconut oil for cooking as it does not turn rancid when heated, even at a high heat.

▶ BEDRIDDEN

If you are bedridden with RA and can barely tolerate noise, let alone trying to chew anything, ask your carer to make you the vegetable puree, grated apple, mashed banana, juices, smoothies, pure water and green tea with pure honey. This regime will not be too hard to tolerate until you are well enough to eat all the food on the menu.

▶ RAPID DECREASE IN INFLAMMATION

If you are in absolute agony and want to drop your pain and inflammation level quickly, eat only pureed vegetables, fresh fruit salads, fruit juices, smoothies, and green tea and pure water.

However, you will lose weight quickly and if you are already thin due to the arthritis, this may not be ideal for you. If you are overweight and can afford to lose many kilos this will be a bonus for you. If you cannot afford to lose any weight, perhaps just follow this particular regime for one or two days per week. When I did this my ESR dropped 31 points and consequently my pain level dropped significantly as well. If you do this and then go straight back on to a Western diet, your ESR and C reactive Protein will increase and so will your pain level. Alternatively, you could go on a water fast for just two days, this will lower your pain level. However, when you are very sick and in a lot of pain you can have detox symptoms that can be a little hard to tolerate.

Through trial and error I have tried just about everything to come up with the following menu but if you want to become well and you follow the regime to the letter, this can work for you too.

▶ BLOOD TESTS

If you have not had recent blood tests taken, try to have them done before you start this diet. Most importantly, request a copy of your blood tests from your doctor every time you have them done. Take control of your health and your body and keep an eye on your blood tests to see the improvements and this will motivate you to keep going. It also empowers you to be in control of something even if it is just your blood tests because when we are very sick, it is difficult to be in control of anything and this can leave us feeling worthless and of no value. The blood tests check your ESR, C reactive protein, FBC and E/LFT. Not many doctors check your rheumatoid factor level anymore as they do not consider this an important test. From one to five percent of people in normal health have a positive RF factor, including people with liver disease and chronic or viral infections. C reactive Protein levels measure the inflammation in your body. When I was very sick, mine was 34, for years now it has been < 4.

If your doctor does not co-operate with you in your efforts to take control of your own health and help you to come off your medication slowly in order for this diet to help you, then please look for another doctor. If your doctor continues to give you that condescending pat on the head, or tries to bully you into continuing the way you have been going—under his control but still sick—then look for another doctor who is just as interested as you are in your efforts to regain your health.

In telling them what I was trying to do, I have had different doctors laugh at me, bully me and treat me with contempt as though I was a child. You need to be strong and to stand up for yourself. I do understand, however, when you are sick with RA, you do not have the energy to take back control over much of anything. If your health is weighing you down too much to seek alternative doctors, just do not go back to the skeptical one. Remember, it is your choice. It is your health.

Many doctors respect patients trying to get themselves well. Doctors are often frustrated with patients who will not stop eating high fat food, never exercise and yet live at the doctor's surgery crying poor health and wondering why they suffer obesity, diabetes and high blood pressure, to name just a few. No wonder some doctors just prescribe medication because they know the patient will not do anything about their own poor health. Most patients will not take responsibility for their own health or, more to the point, their lack of health.

▶ LIQUID HERBAL REMEDIES

Be very careful of liquid herbal remedies as they are usually in an ethanol base, a derivative of alcohol. The ethanol will exacerbate your pain level. Again, I have found out the hard way, because my diet is so basic I can pin point the ingredient in my diet that caused me pain. When I stopped taking these ingredients the pain ceased within a couple of days. Furthermore, you need to be on the lookout for liquid remedies that contain orange and caramel flavors. These also caused me pain because orange is especially high in acid and can increase your pain level. Do not eat any colorings or flavorings.

If you stick to the diet and fresh foods, you will not have to concern yourself with these additives and flavorings. When you buy herbal tablets over the counter, always carefully read the ingredients in everything before you consume them.

▶ CAMPHOR AND PESTICIDES

If you have any camphor blocks or crystals in your home to get rid of moths, please think about throwing them out. I do not have my house sprayed with pesticides, as it is hard enough having to breathe in the toxic chemicals from the pollution in the air we breathe, let alone spraying toxic chemicals straight into my home. I do not use fly sprays and have become an excellent shot with the fly swatter. In addition, I do not have a cupboard full of chemicals to remove stains on everything from clothes, carpet, tiles and walls.

I do not use disinfectants and I do not have a spray for this and a spray for that. I don't even use hair spray or chemical deodorants. I cannot even walk down the supermarket aisle full of detergents and washing powder without it affecting my nose. It usually makes me sneeze. I try to keep everything simple and as natural as possible.

▶ SKIN CARE & DEODORANT

Try and use a natural regime for example, try the Aloe Vera range of products or the Rosehip brand of skin care, which use only organic ingredients. You can find these products in your health food shop along with other good brands. Be wary of perfumes because of their chemical components. Once you become well and your body is detoxified, you will become more sensitive to your environment and you will be able to smell and taste things that you have not experienced in a long time. The strong smell of perfume can be offensive once your sense of taste and smell return. I haven't used chemical perfume in many years. I don't see the point of paying for over priced chemicals to splash all over my body. These chemicals are toxic to your health and our environment. In fact, according to the latest statistics, we spray over two hundred and seventy chemicals on our bodies daily. I use Ylang Ylang on my neck to make me smell nice. It is all natural. You need to be careful what you put on your skin. If you can't eat it, then don't put it on your skin.

I now use organic coconut oil as a face and body moisturizer. To exfoliate your skin, use 2/3 cup of brown sugar and one tablespoon of organic coconut oil. This will leave your skin silky soft, rejuvenate your skin and remove dead skin cells.

(Holzapfel 2003) Alternatively, use 1/2 cup of Uncle Toby's raw traditional oats, 1/4 cup of raw sugar and a little water to exfoliate your skin. It's a little messy (I do it in the shower) but, it really does work, leaving your skin nice and clean. There is nothing more beautiful, than fresh, clean, glowing skin.

▶ ALOE VERA GEL

If you suffer from heat rash every summer and find sometimes it is associated with a fungal infection. Instead of going to the doctors or chemist for more chemicals to put on your body, try using Aloe Vera gel or the natural Aloe Vera leaf from a plant (although it is very sticky and may not be practical), and apply morning and night to the affected area. The rash along with the fungal infection will disappear. Continue to use at least once or twice a week in the hot months to keep it a bay.

I now grow my own Aloe Vera plant and place the gel on sunspots which disappear in a few days to a week. It is great for dry skin and any where on the body. If you slice a piece of the fresh gel, just enough to cover the area, but not the whole thickness of the leaf, and place it over a sun spot, or sore, and let it sit there until the outer part dries out, it will adhere to the skin like a band aid, with the gel underneath healing as nature intended. You will be able to move your arm or leg, without it falling off. Once the aloe is thin like sticky tape, pull it off, as this means the gel has been completely absorbed by your body. Repeat again until the sun spot has completely gone. I also use Aloe Vera Gel under my arms as a natural deodorant. It keeps you smelling fresh all day. You could use a natural plant or bottle for this. Or sometimes I use 100% natural mineral salts. I use the spray bottle, or you could use the stick. Shop bought deodorants from the supermarket, is filled with chemicals and is not conducive to your health.

Furthermore, if you have fresh aloe, peel one or two leaves by slicing down each side to get the sharp side bits of, then fillet the leaf like you would fish, and place the gel with your smoothie into the blender for the last 10 seconds of blending. This is very healing for your digestive tract, and will do wonders for your skin.

▶ INFLAMMATION OF THE EYES

When my eyes were inflamed by the arthritis, I could hardly stand daylight let alone sunlight and were so red they looked awful. The last thing I wanted was the RA to have its way with my eyes, so I went along to the doctor and he wanted me to use cortisone eye drops to reduce the inflammation. I told him I would not use cortisone, as I already knew the dangerous side affects of this chemical drug and I did not want to risk what could happen to my eyes. The doctor was rather abrupt with me because I would not follow his instructions and walked me to the door. Some of the side affects of cortisone include the shortening of life, muscle and adrenal gland atrophy, and thinning of the skin.

I was already using colloidal silver, a natural remedy for sore throats and flu-like infections so I phoned the maker of the product and he told me that colloidal silver would get rid of the inflammation in my eyes. I put two drops of colloidal silver into both eyes morning and night. Within three days, there was a marked improvement and by day four or five, the redness was completely gone. Whenever my eyes started to become inflamed, I used the colloidal silver immediately, before it became worse. However, do not put colloidal gold, colloidal four or any other colloidal metal into your eyes except for colloidal silver. Make sure it is a reputable brand. I use "The Original Colloidal Silver" with the brown and white label by the House of Courtnay (E-mail: csilver@ecig.com.au). I would rather trust my eyes to colloidal silver (a natural product) than cortisone's deadly chemicals. Also if you feel a sore throat coming on, spray the back of your throat with colloidal silver and spray up your nose to reduce inflammation and drink fresh garlic, lemon and honey tea and rest.

▶ **IRRITABLE BOWEL SYNDROME**

I developed irritable bowel syndrome several years ago and believe it was caused through the medication prescribed for me for the arthritis, as most anti-inflammatory agents cause abdominal bleeding and upsets. I have been trying to get rid of it ever since, trying everything from Aloe Vera juice, which is very effective for some people, to Mintec (peppermint oil) but the relief was only temporary. Chinese herbs were also tried but unfortunately, they did not work for me. The symptoms were so debilitating and stressful that I contacted my nutritional medicine doctor to see if she could help me.

She got me onto a product called "Ultra Clear Maintain Plus" a nutritional powder that was designed in the United States specifically for irritable bowel. The effects were immediate. I could not believe the relief after suffering for years. I could actually feel it working. I took the powder, morning and night for two weeks, and then when I had an attack. I was so excited to find something that worked. Over the last two years that I have been taking this product, the symptoms have become less intense and less frequent, making my life a happier one, as the pain and diarrhea depleted my energy levels and prevented me from exercising. It also interfered with my raw juices as on certain occasions, cold food could sometimes bring on an attack. Unfortunately, I discovered they have now put on the label that the product contains vegetable oil and always has. When I was using it, it never stated this on the label. But in saying that, it did give me great relief and if you are suffering, it is certainly worth a try for the short term. I think the benefits far out weigh the amount of vegetable oil you may consume. What has come to light for me recently is that most bowel conditions are caused by the imbalance of flora in the intestines.

However, since I started on organic fruits and vegetables I have noticed a huge difference. When ever I ate commercially grown grapes, within five minutes of eating them, I had stomach pain and diarrhea. Since eating organic grapes, I don't get those symptoms. The chemicals and pesticides sprayed on our food are slowly killing us. No wonder most people are suffering with IBS, including young people. What we are ingesting, is slowly killing us. We run to the doctors for a cure, and pop pills, and yet it's the food we are eating that is causing our health problems. Organic fresh produce is the only way to go. If you are good in the garden try growing your own. I now grow tomatoes, lettuce, basil, Asian greens and Aloe Vera. All organically, I don't put any sprays on them at all.

▶ HOT AND COLD THERAPY FOR PAIN RELIEF

If you have a double kitchen sink, (or improvise) fill up one sink with hot water, as hot as you can stand without burning yourself, and fill the other sink with cold water. Seated on a computer chair with wheels to move easily between sinks, place hands and arms/elbows in hot water for five minutes and then in to the cold water for three minutes. Continue this for twenty minutes to half an hour. This creates extra blood flow to the area, hence, more oxygen to the hands and arms creating less pain. This was a great help for me on really bad days.

In addition, you could use square plastic buckets for your feet and hot and cold packs for your shoulders. My feet and ankles were never affected, and I believe this was because my son at a young age started massaging my feet every night, creating plenty of blood flow, even before I was diagnosed with RA. I believe the power of touch caused my feet not to be affected. My rheumatologist used to shake his head, as he could not get over why my feet and ankles were not painful and swollen. I never had any trouble walking. Therefore, touch and a cuddle are important.

▶ SUPPLEMENTS

I never took any supplements when I was sick and on the recovery diet, except for Zinaxin (a natural green ginger) for pain. I didn't want to take the risk of having an adverse reaction to a product, natural or otherwise, that would interfere with the detoxification process of my body. I recovered simply through diet. Or should I say, my diet allowed my immune system to heal me. Some supplements can be very expensive and synthetic supplements can do the same damage as anti-biotics, for example, killing the good bacteria/flora in the bowel. I know some people who pay a fortune for supplements every month, and yet they never drink water.

Supplements will not save you. In fact, they are expensive. I cannot stress enough to put your money into organic fresh produce and let your immune system heal you. Also, I believe the best way to build bone density is to not take calcium tablets, but to exercise, and eat dark green leafy vegetables. Furthermore, to stay healthy you need to eat a diet high in fresh foods, not supplements. Make sure the fruit and vegetables are genuinely organic, with the organic logo, as organic produce have more vitamin and mineral content than non organic produce. Furthermore, you won't be eating chemical poisons and pesticides that weaken your immune system.

I knew a lady who took Gingko Biloba for many years as prevention for heart attack, because her family had a history of heart disease. She died of bowel cancer in her sixties. She never exercised, was over weight, and her diet was not healthy. Therefore, I cannot stress enough, how important a diet high in fruit, vegetables, pure water and exercise is for optimal health. Supplements will not save you. You will get your vital omega 3, 6 and 9 from your diet as well.

If you want to prevent high blood pressure, eat food high in potassium, especially bananas. Your blood pressure and C reactive protein levels will determine how healthy you are, more so than your cholesterol levels. C reactive protein measures the inflammation level in your body. This is what you want to watch out for, for heart disease. Your blood pressure determines the level of blockage in your arteries.

Dr. Mehmet Oz, author of 'You, The Owners manual' states that it is not genetics that determines poor health, it is your lifestyle choices.

The human body is the best picture of the human soul
Ludwig Wittgenstein

Not all who wander are lost
J.R.R. Tolkein

Chapter 7

—*The Recovery Diet*—

Due to their intolerance of cold food and drinks, the menu may vary a little for irritable bowel sufferers. If you suffer from any allergies then, by all means, omit any food that may upset you.

The recovery diet will also reverse lupus, high blood pressure, and I would even try it for all auto-immune diseases, gastric reflux, constipation, heart disease etc;

The raw/vegan diet will reverse multiple sclerosis, cancer, rheumatoid arthritis and just about any disease known to man. Many people have done it.

What you will need:

> *A positive mental attitude!*
> **Juicer**
> **Blender/Vitamix**
> **Fruit baller**
> **Lettuce/salad spinner**
> **Dehydrator (optional)**
> **Natural skin brush**
> **Chemical free/natural skin care**

Zinaxin (a natural ginger for pain from your health food shop)
Natural tooth paste, soap, shampoo and conditioner
Purified water (I have not drank tap water since 1995)
Natural deodorant (free from aluminum)

▶ JUICING

Never scull juices, as they will go straight to your bladder. Swirl and chew the juice in your mouth for a few seconds so the nutrients are absorbed into the blood stream. Drink fruit juices in the morning and leave vegetable juices till later in the morning or afternoon because vegetable juices are extremely potent.

Drink 2 to 2 1/2 liters of fluids a day. This includes pure water and juices, fruit and salads. Fruit and salads are high water content foods.

During the winter months, leave fruit and vegetables for juicing on the kitchen bench until they come to room temperature. A one or two day fast on pure water or watermelon juice is fabulous for your health and very cleansing. It also speeds up the detoxification process. Alternatively, you could eat grapes for one to two days. Do not juice grapes; they are better eaten as fruit because of the fiber content.

If you can do a one day fast a week on pure water or watermelon juice, it will speed up your healing process and literally add years to your life. Alternatively, do one day on raw food each week.

Always drink juices and eat fruit before meals. Never eat fruit after cooked food or at night because it digests rapidly and cannot pass through the stomach if it is on top of other food that takes longer to digest. Do not eat at least three hours before retiring and try and not eat after 7:30pm at night. The best foods to eat are whole foods, in there natural state like fruit, vegetables, nuts, and seeds. A vegetarian diet truly is the way to a longer and healthier quality of life.

▶ DETOXIFICATION SYMPTOMS

Some of the symptoms you may experience with detoxification could include:

- Headache
- Nausea
- Tiredness and lethargy
- Lower back pain due to the kidneys working overtime
- Dizziness
- Halitosis
- Diarrhea
- Runny nose
- Cold or flu
- Vomiting

You may not suffer any detoxification symptoms at all or just in a mild form. Vomiting is rare. Detoxification symptoms are a good sign because they result from the elimination of toxins. Drink plenty of water to help flush them out of your system. You may also need to rest a little more frequently. However, because you are already sick with RA, you may want to leave the one and two day water or juice fasts until you are feeling better. The two-day fasts can cause you to experience detoxification symptoms, especially when your health is already compromised.

When you are on a juice or water only fast, the toxins at cellular level in your body come down to the bloodstream for elimination and this is what causes the detoxification symptoms. When a bowel motion takes place, the toxins exit the body

When I first went on a two-day water fast, I was quite nauseated. On awakening on the morning of the second day, I thought I was going to vomit so before getting out of bed my children made me a cup of tea and some toast to stave off the symptoms. What I should have eaten was a banana, but I didn't quite know what I was doing at the time. Consequently, I did not last the two days on the fast at that particular time. However, the one day that I was on water only, the cleansing process had already started. The peristalsis of the bowel brought on from eating food the next morning, caused a powerful evacuation due to the fasting.

▶ EXERCISE

Exercise is an integral part of your regime to heal yourself. Start out slowly when you are able, but if you are not used to exercising take it really slowly until you can walk twenty minutes at least three times a week and then over time build up to four of five kilometers three to four times a week. Walking is the best exercise for those of us who have suffered with RA as it causes the least amount of stress on our joints. Avoid jogging, especially on hard surfaces, because you can wear out your hips and knees and you do not want to place any stress on your joints that may have already been damaged by the arthritis. Alternatively, you could jump on a re-bounder (mini trampoline) for a minute several times a day and slowly build up to 10 minutes 3 times a day.

If you suffer from irritable bowel syndrome, please do not drink the juices or the cold fruit if they upset you. Please drink the warm teas, and eat the warm food instead. Alternatively, bring the fruit to room temperature before eating. Omit any foods that you already know upset you until you are stronger.

When the menu calls for honey, please use the pure raw unheated honey from the health food shop. My favorite is Yellow Box as it is a light honey. If this is unavailable, use natural bush honey; it may have been heated but it is not full of sugar. Please do not use commercial supermarket blended honey. Do not use packaged or canned foods and always use fresh lemons, not bottled lemon juice. Some other checkpoint areas include:

- Only eat the food on the menu.
- No coffee, tea or foods that contain caffeine.
- No dried fruits that are not organic as they may contain sulphur, vegetable oil and preservatives.
- The organically dried apricots are black. Do not buy the orange ones.
- You will need organic coconut oil, apricot oil and cold pressed extra virgin olive oil. I prefer the apricot oil as it is such a light oil.

- Everything must be fresh including garlic as the bottled garlic has vinegar in it and may exacerbate your pain.
- Purified water.
- Remember, people who eat sparingly live longer.
- Use green apples for juicing.
- Consume all juices within 15 minutes or they will start to oxidize (lose oxygen) unless you have an expensive juicer that retains the enzymes for a couple of days.

If you also suffer from diabetes, omit the juices and fruit where necessary and eat more warm foods and salads. Please check with your doctor, who is a nutritional medicine practitioner, and supportive of what you are doing to help you lower your dose of insulin or tablets.

Should you need to use a little salt, use only Celtic grey sea salt or Himalayan salt. I use Willow Vale Organics as I find it the tastiest. Do not be put off by its light grey color, which is due to the minerals it contains; you can obtain it from the health food shop, or the health food section at the supermarket. Try to use it sparingly. Do not use table salt as it is harmful to your health, and contains aluminum as a flowing agent.

The purines in some vegetables exacerbate gouty arthritis because of the high acid content, which will increase your pain. Please note that *the following fruit and vegetables are not to be eaten* on the recovery diet:

    Apple cider vinegar
    Balsamic vinegar
    All vinegars

- Asparagus
- Butter
- Capsicum
- Chilies
- Grapefruit
- Mandarin
- Margarine
- Tangelo
- Oranges
- Pineapple
- Spices
- Spinach
- Dairy
- Meat
- Seafood
- Flesh
- Chicken

If you stick to the food on the menu, you will not have to worry about what you can and cannot have. If you can try to drink nothing but watermelon juice till lunch time for two or three weeks you will be doing yourself and your bowel a big favor. Even if you do it once or twice a week, it will speed up the detoxification process. If you continue to smoke or drink alcohol, there are no guarantees that this diet will work for you.

I have allowed extra food on the menu at meal times because people on Western diets are accustomed to eating more food, especially men. However, I cannot eat everything on the menu at one sitting because highly nutritious food is very filling. I am used to small meals and feel very satisfied. Remember, people who eat sparingly live longer.

If you can go without bread altogether it is more beneficial as many people are wheat intolerant.

Don't eat after 7:30pm at night. You will also find that you will no longer suffer from heart burn. Heart burn can eventually lead to cancer of the esophagus.

It is not the mountain we conquer, but ourselves
Sir Edmund Hillary

**We shall draw from the heart of suffering itself
the means of inspiration and survival**
Sir Winston Churchill

The following diet was my original diet that made me well. However I have since moved on to becoming a 100% raw/vegan, eating only raw, living organic food, which allows the body to heal faster and give you optimal health.

The raw food diet is also included in this book. You choose which way to go. Perhaps you could do this diet first to help you transition over to the raw food diet at a later stage if you so choose.

Chapter 8

—*The recovery diet seven day menu*—

Please read the preceding information before starting this diet

DAY ONE—MONDAY

BREAKFAST

Watermelon juice, or cup of fresh lemon tea with honey, or glass of pure water.
1 or 2 ripe bananas, or fruit salad, or fruit smoothie, see recipe
Cup of herb tea with honey (green tea is excellent.)

MORNING TEA

Watermelon juice, or cup of herb tea
Fruit

LUNCH

Watermelon juice, or water, drink before food

Platter of fresh fruit and fresh raw vegetables (carrot sticks, broccoli, cauliflower, mushroom, and zucchini) with home made hummus. See recipe

Cup of herb tea

AFTERNOON TEA

Carrot and apple juice/fresh rock melon/grapes/bananas

DINNER

Salad with apricot oil dressing (see recipe)

Steamed vegetables. Squeeze over a little fresh lemon juice for flavor, and or a little honey is really nice. Sweet potato, pumpkin, cauliflower, broccoli, carrots, zucchini or whatever vegetables you like.

Cup of herb tea

SUPPER

Cup of herb tea

RECOVERY DIET
DAY TWO—TUESDAY

BREAKFAST

Watermelon juice, or water, or cup of fresh lemon tea with honey

Fruit salad, or fruit and nut smoothie, see recipe

Cup of herb tea

MORNING TEA

Watermelon juice, or water

Dried organic raisins, and a few walnuts

Banana

LUNCH

Watermelon juice, or water. Drink before food

Large vegetable salad, with apricot oil/olive oil dressing. (See recipe)

Banana

Cup of herb tea

AFTERNOON TEA

Carrot and apple juice/beetroot and apple juice, 1/4 cup of chemical free almonds.

DINNER
Large vegetable salad with avocado dressing (See recipe)
Banana
Cup of herb tea

SUPPER
Cup of herb tea

RECOVERY DIET
DAY THREE—WEDNESDAY

BREAKFAST

Watermelon juice, or water, or fresh lemon tea with honey. Banana, or smoothie, see recipe

Pureed vegetables, see recipe

Cup of herb tea

MORNING TEA

Watermelon juice/cup of herb tea

Dried organic sultanas

Chemical free almonds

LUNCH

Watermelon juice, drink before food

Organic spelt bread salad sandwich with avocado, used instead of butter or margarine. (See recipe)

Cup of herb tea

AFTERNOON TEA

Carrot, fresh ginger and apple juice/beetroot, celery and apple juice

Sunflower seeds and sesame seeds

Raw unsalted cashews (a small handful)

DINNER
Vegetable soup
Banana
Cup of herb tea

SUPPER
Cup of herb tea

THE RECOVERY DIET
DAY FOUR-THURSDAY

BREAKFAST

Watermelon juice, or fresh lemon tea with honey, or water
Large fruit salad and bananas, or fruit smoothie, see recipe

MORNING TEA

Watermelon juice, or water. Drink before food
Dried organic apricots and a handful of walnuts
Banana

LUNCH

Watermelon juice, or water, drink before food
Brown rice salad (see recipe)
Cup of herb tea

AFTERNOON TEA

Carrot and apple juice/beetroot and apple juice
Dried organic currants/apricots/sultanas
Chemical free almonds

DINNER

Dry baked potato, pumpkin, sweet potato (no oil)
Steamed vegetables, pour over a little lemon juice if desired
Cup of herb tea

SUPPER

Cup of herb tea

THE RECOVERY DIET
DAY FIVE-FRIDAY

BREAKFAST
Watermelon juice, or fresh lemon tea with honey
Vegetable soup (see recipe)
Cup of herb tea

MORNING TEA
Watermelon juice, or cup of herb tea
Fruit

LUNCH
Watermelon juice, or water, drink before food
Vegetable soup (see recipe) and or salad
Banana
Cup of herb tea

AFTERNOON TEA
Carrot, ginger and apple juice
Fruit

DINNER
Watermelon juice, or water, drink before food
Salad
Dry grilled vegetables (see recipe)
Banana
Cup of herb of tea

SUPPER
Cup of herb tea

THE RECOVERY DIET
DAY SIX-SATURDAY

BREAKFAST

Watermelon juice, or fresh lemon tea with honey

Fruit salad, banana, or fruit smoothie, (see recipe)

Vegetable soup

Cup of herb tea

MORNING TEA

Watermelon juice, or cup of herb tea

Dried organic fruit

Banana

Cup of herb tea

LUNCH

Watermelon juice

Pureed vegetables

Banana

Cup of herb tea

AFTERNOON TEA

Carrot, ginger and apple juice, or beetroot and apple juice

Fruit

DINNER
Salad with tarragon and garlic dressing (see recipe)
Steamed vegetables, with brown rice with a squeeze of lemon juice and or honey (optional)
Cup of herb tea

SUPPER
Cup of herb tea

THE RECOVERY DIET
DAY SEVEN-SUNDAY

BREAKFAST
Watermelon juice, or fresh lemon tea with honey
Vegetable soup (see recipe) fruit smoothie, (see recipe)
Cup of herb tea

MORNING TEA
Watermelon juice, or cup of herb tea
Fruit

LUNCH
Watermelon juice, drink before food
Large vegetable salad with apricot oil/olive oil dressing (see recipe)
Banana

AFTERNOON TEA
Carrot and apple juice/beetroot and apple juice
1/4 cup of chemical free almonds

DINNER
Large vegetable salad with avocado dressing (see recipe)
Banana
Cup of herb tea

SUPPER
Cup of herb tea

THE RECOVERY DIET
AN EXTRA DAY
DAY EIGHT

BREAKFAST

Fruit smoothie, (see recipe)

MORNING TEA

Fruit salad (see recipe)

Sultanas (only organic) (not sultanas soaked in vegetable oil and sulphur

LUNCH

Watermelon juice

Whole meal lavish bread salad roll up (see recipe)

Cup of herb tea

AFTERNOON TEA

Carrot and apple juice/beetroot and apple juice

Fresh carrot sticks dipped into hummus/avocado dip (see recipe)

DINNER

Pumpkin and Lentil soup

Banana

Cup of herb tea

SUPPER

Cup of herb tea

Obstacles are those frightful things you see when you take your eyes off your goal.

Henry Ford

We are what we repeatedly do.

Aristotle

Chapter 9

—*Recipes recovery diet*—

- **ROCKMELON AND BANANA ICE CREAM**

1/2 fresh frozen rock melon
4 fresh frozen bananas
1/2-1 cup of juiced rock melon.

Thaw frozen fruit for a few minutes on the kitchen bench without thawing completely, then cube into small pieces and place in the blender. Pour some of the rock melon juice into the blender and blend. Use more rock melon juice if needed to facilitate blending.

- **ROCKMELON AND BANANA SMOOTHIE**

1/4 rock melon
2 bananas.

Place rock melon and bananas in blender until smooth.

- **MANGO AND BANANA SMOOTHIE**

1 mango
1 banana
A little water to facilitate blending.

Place fruit into the blender until smooth.

- **BERRY PROTEIN SMOOTHIE**

1/4 cup blueberries
1/2 cup fresh/frozen mixed berries
1 large banana
1/8 cup almonds
1 dessertspoon organic sunflower seeds.
2 teaspoons of organic flaxseeds.

Place in blender and blend until smooth.

- **MANGO AND BANANA ICE CREAM**

2 frozen mangos
1-2 frozen bananas.

Place fruit on the kitchen bench and allow thawing for a few minutes and then slice. Place ingredients into the blender until thick and creamy.

- **FRESH LEMON TEA WITH HONEY**

1 cup of boiling water
1 fresh lemon
Raw pure unheated honey/natural bush honey

Pour water into cup and squeeze in lemon juice and 1-1 1/2 teaspoons honey.

- **FRESH GARLIC AND LEMON TEA**

2 fresh cloves garlic
1 lemon
1-2 teaspoons honey.

Slice garlic into large pieces and place in bottom of cup. Pour in boiling water and squeeze in 1/4 of juiced lemon and honey. Steep for 5 minutes, stir and drink slowly. This is a natural remedy for sore throats, colds and flu. Garlic is natures anti-biotic and it tastes great.

- **FLAXSEED MIX** (See raw/vegan diet)

Grind with a coffee grinder, 2 Table spoons of each
Organic Flax seeds
Organic Sunflower seeds
Organic Pepitos (pumpkin seeds)
Organic white sesame seeds

Mix powdered mixture together and store in the fridge.

Put 2 table spoons of mixture in your green smoothie, every day.
This will make enough for a about week. Don't make too much, it's best to keep it as fresh as possible. If you have the time, grind the mix, fresh every day. This mix will provide you with your daily omega 3, 6, & 9s.

- **FRUIT SALAD**

6-8 fresh cherries/frozen cherries
6-8 watermelon balls
6-8 rock melon balls
2 kiwi fruit
1 green apple cut up
1 banana
8 blueberries fresh/frozen
1 passion fruit

Place fruit into a bowl and pour over watermelon juice. Do not use orange juice because of the acid content. Allow frozen cherries/blueberries (no additives/flavorings/sugar) to come to room temperature.

- **SALAD**

Lettuce
Cucumber
Bok Choy
Tomato
Onion
Sprouts
1 fresh lemon

Cold pressed extra virgin olive oil/cold pressed apricot oil. 1-1 & 1/2 caps of oil only. Keep your fat content to 10% of your diet, including nuts.

Celtic sea salt
Tarragon.

Wash and dry lettuce, then cut up all ingredients and place in a bowl. Squeeze over lemon juice, oil and a little salt. Use any vegetable or salad ingredient you like. Never use apple cider vinegar; it gave me terrible pain because of the acid content. Only use fresh lemon juice.

- **SALSA**

1 tomato
1/2 small onion
1/4 Lebanese cucumber
1 green capsicum
1 clove of fresh garlic
1/4 fresh lemon
Fresh basil leaves
Celtic sea salt
1 Tbs cold pressed extra virgin olive oil.

Dice ingredients into bite size pieces and place in a bowl. Stir and squeeze over lemon juice, olive oil, salt and herbs.

- **WHOLEMEAL SALAD SANDWICH**

Two slices of good quality whole meal bread/organic spelt bread preferably (has no vegetable oil or preservatives), avocado

Lettuce
Tomato
Onion
Bok Choy
Cucumber
Alfalfa sprouts.
Fresh grated beetroot (not canned)

You can use the bread fresh or have it lightly toasted. Spread some avocado over the bread instead of butter and then layer the rest of the ingredients, slicing the bok choy in thin strips. Slice in two, or quarters.

- **WHOLEMEAL LAVISH BREAD ROLL UP**

1 piece of whole meal lavish bread
Avocado
Tomato
Lettuce
Onion
Cucumber
Sprouts
Carrots
Bok Choy/Kale
Fresh grated beetroot

Lay out the lavish bread and spread with avocado (no butter) place on cut up ingredients, thinly slice the bok choy and roll up and serve. Or you can place all ingredients into a lettuce leaf and roll, instead. The less bread you consume the better.

- **LARGE VEGETABLE SALAD**

Dark lettuce
Onion
Tomato
Cucumber
Grated carrot
Bok choy
Broccoli sprigs
Organic sunflower seeds
Organic sesame seeds
Cauliflower florets.
Your favorite sprouts

Separate lettuce, wash and spin dry in the lettuce spinner as wet lettuce will go limp once the oil is added. Place lettuce in a mixing bowl with the other cut up ingredients and any sprouts you like. Pour over apricot or avocado dressing. Do not use apple cider vinegar only use lemon juice

- **LARGE WARM WINTER SALAD**

Lettuce
Onion
Tomato
Cucumber
Carrots
Broccoli sprigs
Bok choy
Zucchini
Cauliflower florets.

Slice the broccoli sprigs, carrots, cauliflower and zucchini vegetables into bite size bits and steam for 5 minutes then toss through with the other cut up fresh salad ingredients. Pour over avocado dressing. Do not use apple cider vinegar, only use lemon juice.

- **PUREED VEGETABLES**

1 large sweet potato
4 large carrots
4 large slices of pumpkin
1/4 cauliflower
Small head of broccoli
1 cup of fresh green beans
2 large onions
4 cloves of garlic

1 & 1/2 cups of water
1 Tsp. dried parsley
1 Tsp. dried Tarragon

Use fresh herbs if you have them. Also, use your favorite herbs. These quantities make enough for several days.

Peel and chop vegetables into large cubes and place in a large saucepan with water and herbs. Cover and bring to the boil. Simmer for about twenty minutes or until tender. Place all ingredients in a blender and puree. Serve with a little Celtic sea salt. This is great if your jaw is too painful to masticate food.

- **VEGETABLE SOUP**

1/2 zucchini
1 large sweet potato
4 large carrots
1/2 large pumpkin
1/4-1/2 cauliflower
Small head of broccoli
1 cup of fresh green beans
6 Brussels sprouts
2 large onions
4 cloves of garlic
1 liter of water
1 Tsp. dried parsley
1 Tsp. dried tarragon

Use fresh/favorite herbs if you have them. Quantities make enough for several days; store half in the freezer and the rest in the refrigerator.

Peel and chop vegetables into small cubes and place in a large saucepan with water and herbs. Bring to the boil and simmer for 40-50 minutes. Allow the pumpkin to melt down into the soup for more flavor. Serve with a little Celtic sea salt. Please use the sea salt sparingly. Try any vegetable you like but not spinach or asparagus, as they contain purines, which can exacerbate arthritis pain, especially gout.

- **DRY GRILLED VEGETABLES**

1 zucchini
1 tomato
4 mushrooms
1 left over steamed potato
1 left over steamed pumpkin left over carrots
Sesame seeds
Juice of fresh lemon (optional).

Slice zucchini in halves length ways, slice tomato in half and place in a moderately hot pan or on the grill with other vegetables and grill until brown, turning once. Serve on a plate and squeeze over lemon juice if desired and sesame seeds. Serves 1

- **DRY BAKED VEGETABLES**

Potatoes
Pumpkin
Carrots
Onion
Sweet potato.

Peel and cut up vegetables. Steam for 10 minutes except onion and then place on an oven tray and put into a hot oven, preheated at 200 degrees, for about 45 minutes or until cooked. Turn once. Steaming the vegetables first will make the vegetables crispier. Serve with green beans, or vegetables of your choice.

- **PUMPKIN AND LENTIL SOUP**

¾ Jap/kent pumpkin
1/2 Large cauli
6 Large carrots
1 & 1/2 cups of brown lentils
6 Cloves of garlic
2 Large onions
Parsley (fresh/dried)
Tarragon (fresh/dried)
Pinch Celtic Sea Salt

Place chopped up vegetables and herbs in a large saucepan with 2 liters of water. Bring to the boil, and simmer until lentils are tender, about 45 minutes-1 hour.

Place ¾ of soup in blender and puree, leaving some lentils (not vegetables) to mix in for some texture. Should last a week. Freeze half and save for later.

- **DRY BAKED STUFFED CAPSICUM**

1 large capsicum
1/2 cup cooked organic brown rice
1 tomato chopped
1/2 cooked zucchini
1/2 small cooked onion
1 tsp dried basil

1 fresh clove garlic (optional)
Celtic sea salt

Cut the top of the capsicum and scoop out seeds. Dice tomato, garlic, zucchini, and slice onion. Brown the tomato, garlic, zucchini and onion in a frying pan with the brown rice. Add in salt, basil and squeeze over a little lemon juice. Place mixture into the capsicum until full and place lid on capsicum. Place into a hot oven at 180 degrees for about 20-30 minutes until capsicum is tender and a little brown.

Serve on a plate with a little olive oil mixed with a squeeze of lemon juice drizzled over the capsicum. Serve with a salad.

- **WALNUT STIR FRY**

1/2 cup walnuts
1 diced zucchini
4 diced yellow squash
1 diced small onion
2 Tbs. cold pressed organic, extra virgin coconut oil
Fresh basil
Celtic sea salt.

Pour oil in pan and bring to low heat. Stir-fry zucchini, squash and onion until tender. Sprinkle in a little basil and salt. Add walnuts at the end and stir through. Serve.

- **AVOCADO SALAD**

1/2 an avocado
Tomato
Cucumber
Onion
Lettuce
1/8 cup of raw cashews.

Cube the avocado and place in a bowl with the cut up salad ingredients and cashews. Toss through and pour over avocado dressing. Serves 1

• WALNUT SALAD

Lettuce
1 tomato
6 slices cucumber
Onion
Fresh or dried herbs of your choice (no spices)
1/4 cup organic dried raisins or
Organic sultanas
1/8 cup of walnuts.

Wash, dry, and separate lettuce, dice tomato and place in a bowl with other salad ingredients including the raisins/sultanas and walnuts. Toss through with herbs, serve and pour over apricot or olive oil dressing.

• BROWN RICE SALAD

2-3 cups of cooked organic brown rice
2 shallots sliced
2 fresh corn cobs, cut corn off cob
3 tomatoes
1/2 Lebanese cucumber
1/2 cup organic sultanas
1/8 cup olive oil
1 fresh lemon
Fresh/dried tarragon
Parsley

Pinch Celtic sea salt

Mix all ingredients together, squeeze over lemon juice, salt, oil and serve.

DRESSINGS AND DIPS

- **APRICOT OIL DRESSING**

1/2 to 1 Tbs apricot oil
Squeeze of lemon juice
Garlic optional

Celtic sea salt (must be a light grey in color) I use Willow Vale brand.
Pour apricot oil over salad and then the lemon juice. Toss for a beautiful light taste. If you prefer a stronger taste, use a good cold pressed extra virgin olive oil.

- **AVOCADO DRESSING**

1 large avocado
1/4-1/2 of a juiced lemon
Celtic sea salt
Olive oil/apricot oil
1 Tsp. honey

Mash the avocado and pour in lemon juice, oil and honey, mix in and pour over salad. Make it up to the required consistency to suit your taste.

- **TARRAGON GARLIC DRESSING**

1 clove garlic
1 lemon
1-2 Tbs cold pressed extra virgin olive oil (organic if you can)
Celtic sea salt
1 tsp. dried tarragon
1-2 t honey
Little pure water.

Crush garlic clove into a bowl and add a squeeze of lemon to taste, add oil, honey, sea salt, tarragon (fresh herbs if you like). If necessary, add a little water if the lemon juice is too tart or strong. Pour over salad.

- **ITALIAN DRESSING**

1/4 cup of cold pressed olive oil
1 clove garlic
Juiced lemon
Pinch Celtic sea salt
1/2 tsp. dried basil/fresh basil
Little pure water.

Crush garlic in a bowl, Add oil, salt, basil, lemon juice. Pour over salad.

- **HOMMUS**

1 cup of fresh organic chick peas
1/2 cup tahini
2 cloves of fresh garlic
1/2 cup Olive oil
Chives
Juice of 1 lemon
Little pure water

Celtic sea salt. (Do not use normal table salt. Never use pepper)
Soak overnight fresh chickpeas and drain, then place in blender with tahini, garlic, lemon juice, oil and a pinch of salt. Blend on slow speed until you reach the desired consistency. If it is too thick, use a little pure water to help the blending. Add more lemon juice if desired to suit your taste. Hummus is great for dipping raw vegetables. If you want to use hummus for a salad dressing, dilute it with more lemon juice and or pure water. Garnish with chives.

Author's Note

This diet regime worked for me and it may work for you. It is certainly worth a try.

The idea is to eat anti-inflammatory foods, such as fresh fruit and vegetables.

Once you are pain and symptom free, you can then go onto the maintenance regime. If your pain returns, however, omit the offending food. If you introduce one food at a time, you will notice which foods that may trigger an attack.

This diet could take 3-12 months to recover your health. If you eat anything off the menu, you may need to start all over again, as you could undo the healing process with Western diet food. If you continue to smoke or drink alcohol, there is no guarantee this will work.

Dreams are more important than knowledge.
Albert Einstein

**Whatever you can do or dream you can, begin it.
Boldness has genius, power, and magic in it**
Johann Wolfgang Von Goethe

Chapter 10

—*Maintenance diet*—

BREAKFAST IDEAS

- Watermelon juice.
- Fresh lemon tea with honey.
- Rock melon and banana smoothie—See recipe.
- Berry protein smoothie.
- Mango and banana smoothie.
- Mango and banana ice cream.
- Fruit salad or a bowl of grapes.
- Banana ice cream—see recipe.
- Toasted organic spelt (pumpkin, olive or sesame is nice) bread with avocado.
- Mashed banana on spelt toast.
- Grilled tomato, zucchini, eggplant, mushrooms and capsicum. After serving, drizzle over a little cold pressed extra virgin olive oil, lemon juice, basil and a little Celtic sea salt.
- Toasted organic spelt bread with avocado, sliced tomato and a sprinkle of basil.

- Toasted organic spelt bread with hummus, sliced tomato and a sprinkle of basil.
- Vegetable soup with a pinch of marigold Swiss Vegetable Bouillon powder (contains traces of peanuts if you are allergic, please do not use it—if not, it is very tasty). Available at health food shops—See recovery diet recipe for vegetable soup recipe.
- Pureed vegetables with a pinch of marigold Swiss Vegetable Bouillon powder—See recovery diet for recipe.
- Home made or bought organic fresh muesli (not toasted) with fruit. Pour over fresh apple or orange juice.
- Steamed vegetables.

LUNCH IDEAS

- Watermelon juice.
- Platter of fresh fruit and fresh vegetables with hummus or avocado dip—see recipe.
- Avocado and salad sandwich on spelt whole meal bread.
- Whole meal lavish salad roll up.
- Avocado salad.
- Walnut salad.
- Warm winter salad.
- Large vegetable salad.
- Salsa with toasted crunchy whole meal pita bread—See recipe.
- Greek salad with goat's feta cheese—See recipe.
- Toasted spelt bread with goat's feta cheese, avocado, and tomato—See recipe.

- Grilled vegetables with a salad.
- Grilled vegetable burger—see recipe.
- Pureed vegetables with a little bouillon and salad.
- Steamed vegetables.
- Dry baked potato and pumpkin with a salad or home made salsa—See recipe.
- Cucumber and yoghurt salad with crunchy whole meal pita bread—See recipe.
- Brown rice stir fry—See recipe.

DINNER IDEAS

- Watermelon juice.
- Dry baked stuffed capsicum/eggplant—See recipe.
- Avocado salad—See recipe.
- Steamed vegetables with salsa dressings—See recipe.
- Pureed vegetables with a salad.
- Grilled vegetables with pesto dressing—See recipe.
- Baked potato, pumpkin, sweet potato and carrots, cooked in organic coconut oil
- Large salad of your choice.
- Large raw vegetable platter with hummus/avocado dressing/home made pesto—See recipe.
- Steamed vegetables and or a salad, with one of the dressings shown.
- Grilled vegetable burgers with salad—See recipe.
- Whole meal organic spelt pasta served with char grilled vegetables or tomato pesto—See recipe.

- Idaho potatoes served with natural goat's milk yoghurt, chopped chives and a salad.
- Whole meal organic spelt and vegetable pasta with mashed steamed pumpkin, chopped chives and a little grated feta cheese (goats).
- Cucumber and yoghurt salad with crunchy whole meal pita bread—See recipe.
- Brown rice stir—fry—See recipe.
- Large warm winter salad—See recipe.
- Walnut stir fry—see recipe.

RECIPES MAINTENANCE DIET

- **FRESH LEMON TEA WITH HONEY**

1 cup of boiling water
1 fresh lemon
Raw, pure, unheated honey—natural bush honey.

Pour water into cup and squeeze in lemon juice and 1-1 1/2 teaspoons honey.

- **FRESH GARLIC AND LEMON TEA**

2 fresh cloves garlic
1 lemon
1-2 teaspoons honey.

Slice garlic into pieces and place into bottom of cup. Pour in boiling water and squeeze in 1/4 of juiced lemon and honey. Steep for 5 minutes, stir and drink slowly. This is a natural remedy for sore throats, colds and flu. Garlic is a natural anti-biotic and it tastes great. You may not have any friends left after drinking garlic and lemon tea, but you will be healthier.

- **BANANA ICE CREAM**

4 fresh frozen bananas

1/4 cup of orange juice—use only enough orange juice to facilitate blending.

Thaw frozen bananas for a few minutes on the kitchen bench and then slice. Place into blender and add orange juice slowly to make ice cream. Too much juice will make it too runny. If orange juice still causes you too much acid and pain, use freshly squeezed apple juice.

- **ROCKMELON AND BANANA ICE CREAM**

1/2 a fresh frozen rock melon
4 fresh frozen bananas
1/2-1 cup of juiced rock melon.

Thaw fruit for a few minutes on the kitchen bench then cube into small pieces and place in the blender. Pour some of the rock melon juice into the blender and blend. Use more rock melon juice if needed to facilitate blending.

- **ROCKMELON AND BANANA SMOOTHIE**

1/4 rock melon
2 bananas.

Place rock melon and bananas in blender until smooth.

- **MANGO AND BANANA SMOOTHIE**

2 large mangos
1-2 bananas.

Place fruit into the blender until smooth.

- **BERRY PROTEIN SMOOTHIE**

1/2 cup blueberries
1/2 cup raspberries (fresh/frozen mixed berries maybe used)
1 banana
1/4 cup almonds
1 dessertspoon organic sunflower seeds.
2 teaspoons organic flaxseeds.
Place in blender and blend until smooth.

- **MANGO AND BANANA ICE CREAM**

2 frozen mangos
1-2 frozen bananas.

Place fruit on the kitchen bench and allow thawing for a few minutes and then slice. Place ingredients into the blender until thick and creamy.

Place mangos and bananas in blender until smooth.

• DRY BAKED STUFFED CAPSICUM

1 large capsicum/eggplant
1/2 cup cooked organic brown rice
1 tomato
1/2 zucchini
1/2 small onion
1 tsp. dried basil
1 fresh clove garlic (optional)
Celtic sea salt
Lemon juice
Olive oil.

Cut the top of the capsicum and scoop out seeds. Dice tomato, garlic, zucchini, and slice onion. Brown the tomato, garlic, zucchini and onion in a frying pan with the brown rice. Add in salt, basil and squeeze over a little lemon juice. Place mixture into the capsicum until full and place lid on capsicum. Place into a hot oven at 180 degrees for about 20-30 minutes until capsicum is tender and a little brown.

Serve on a plate with a little olive oil mixed with a squeeze of lemon juice drizzled over the capsicum. Serve with a salad.

• WALNUT STIR FRY

1/2 cup walnuts
1 diced zucchini
4 cut up yellow squash
1 diced small onion

2 Tbs. cold pressed extra virgin olive oil
Fresh basil
Celtic sea salt.

Pour oil in pan and bring to low heat. Stir-fry zucchini, squash and onion until tender. Sprinkle in a little basil and salt. Add walnuts at the end and stir through. Serve.

- **LARGE WARM WINTER SALAD**

Lettuce
Onion
Tomato
Cucumber
Carrots
Broccoli sprigs
Zucchini
Cauliflower florets.

Slice the vegetables into bite size bits and steam for 5 minutes then toss through with the other cut up salad ingredients. Pour over avocado dressing.

- **SALSA**

1 tomato
1/2 small onion

1/4 Lebanese cucumber
1 green capsicum
1 clove of fresh garlic
1/4 fresh lemon
Fresh basil leaves
Celtic sea salt
1 Tbs cold pressed extra virgin olive oil.

Dice ingredients into bite size pieces and place in a bowl. Stir and squeeze over lemon juice, olive oil, salt and herbs.

- **GREEK SALAD WITH GOAT FETTA CHEESE**

Lettuce
1 tomato
6 slices of Lebanese cucumber
1/4 small onion
1/4 cup of sliced pitted black olives
Goat feta cheese.

Wash and dry lettuce and break into a salad bowl, cut up salad ingredients and place in the bowl. Sprinkle over olives and a little cheese. Pour over Italian dressing and toss.

- **CUCUMBER AND YOGHURT SALAD**

1/2 Lebanese cucumber
2 cloves garlic
1/2 jar goat's milk natural yoghurt.

Cut up cucumber into small pieces and place into a bowl. Crush garlic into garlic crusher or dice up into very small pieces and add to cucumber. Pour over yoghurt and stir. Cover and place into fridge for a couple of hours for the flavors to blend. Serve with whole meal pita bread or with a salad.

- **GOATS FETTA CHEESE AND AVOCADO ON TOAST**

1 slice of olive organic/white/whole meal spelt bread
Goat feta cheese
Avocado
Tomato
Fresh basil.

Toast bread and leave until dried and crunchy. Spread over a little goat's cheese then, spread over a little avocado and place tomato slices of top. Sprinkle over fresh basil and serve.

• GRILLED VEGETABLE BURGER

1 whole meal roll
1 vegetable pattie (see recipe)
Sliced tomato
Sliced onion
Lettuce
Avocado dressing

Spread roll with avocado, heat vegetable burger on grill and place on roll, cover with tomato slices, onion, lettuce and avocado dressing.

• GRILLED VEGETABLE PATTIES

3 large potatoes
2 fresh corn cobs
1 large grated carrot
4 grated broccoli sprigs
4 grated cauliflower sprigs
1/2 zucchini grated
1 small onion diced, (optional)
1/2 cup fresh blended whole meal/spelt breadcrumbs,
Celtic sea salt
Parsley
Tarragon
2 organic/ free range eggs.

Steam the potatoes until cooked and mash into a large bowl. Scrape the corn of the cobs and add to potatoes with the carrot, broccoli, cauliflower, onion, breadcrumbs, salt, herbs and the eggs. Mix into patties and roll into breadcrumbs then place in the fridge for at least 30 minutes. Take out of the fridge and let stand for 5-10 minutes then bake in the oven at 180 degrees until brown on both sides approximately 40 minutes. Or cook in organic coconut oil until brown on both sides. (Organic Coconut oil is the only oil that does not turn rancid when heated) Serve with a salad or on a whole meal bun.

- **BROWN RICE STIR FRY**

2 cups of boiled organic brown rice
1 large onion diced
1 large tomato cut into pieces
1 small zucchini cubes
6 mushrooms diced
1 fresh lemon
Fresh basil
Celtic sea salt
Cold pressed extra virgin olive oil.

Place rice in a pan without oil, and brown. Meanwhile using another pan, brown onions, tomato, mushrooms and zucchini, adding the salt and a little lemon juice to facilitate steaming. When the vegetables are cooked mix in with the rice and serve. Drizzle over some lemon juice, olive oil and Celtic sea salt.

- **WHOLEMEAL PASTA & CHARGRILLED VEGETABLES**

1/2 packet whole meal pasta/organic spelt pasta/vegetable pasta, Celtic sea salt
1 capsicum
1/2 eggplant
1 zucchini
2 tomatoes
3 small squashes
Grated parmesan cheese/goats feta cheese/raw cheese from a grass fed jersey cow if you can get it.
Fresh basil
Parsley
Virgin olive oil.

Place pasta into boiling salted water. Cook until tender and then drain. Meanwhile, place all vegetables in the oven or on a grill until roasted. Cut cooked vegetables into chunks and stir through cooked pasta with herbs. Drizzle over oil, lemon juice and a little salt. Serves 2

- **PUMPKIN PASTA**

1/2 packet whole meal pasta/organic spelt pasta
Celtic sea salt
1/4 large pumpkin
Goat feta cheese.

Boil pasta in boiling salted water until tender and then drain. Meanwhile, steam pumpkin until tender. Mash cooked pumpkin and spread over pasta in bowl. Sprinkle a little cheese on top and serve.

- **IDAHO POTATOES**

2 large Pontiac potatoes
Goats milk natural yoghurt
Chopped chives.

Wash potatoes and place in the oven without peeling at 200 degrees for about 30-40 minutes or until cooked. Cut in halves and place on a plate. Spoon over a little yoghurt, and sprinkle with chives. Serve with steamed vegetables or a salad.

DRESSINGS AND DIPS

- **AVOCADO DIP**

2 Large avocados
1 organic egg
1/4 cup juiced lemon
1 Tbs olive oil
1-2 tsp. sweet chili sauce
Celtic sea salt
Dijon mustard (optional)

Mash the avocados in with the oil and egg, lemon juice, sweet chili sauce and salt.

Instead of salt, you could use a pinch of marigold Swiss Vegetable Bouillon powder. You could also add a little curry powder for a change.

- **APRICOT OIL DRESSING**

1/2-1 Tbs. apricot oil
Squeeze of lemon juice

Pour apricot oil over salad and then the lemon juice. Toss for a beautiful light taste. If you prefer a stronger taste, use a good cold pressed extra virgin olive oil.

- **AVOCADO DRESSING**

1 avocado
Pinched Cayenne pepper
1/4-1/2 of a juiced lemon
Celtic sea salt
1 tsp. honey.

Mash the avocado and pour in lemon juice and honey, mix well to a consistency that suits, and pour over the salad.

- **TARRAGON GARLIC DRESSING**

1 clove garlic
1 lemon
1-2 Tbs. cold pressed extra virgin olive oil (organic if you can)
Celtic sea salt
1 tsp. dried tarragon
1-2 tsp. honey
Little pure water
Dijon mustard (optional)

Crush garlic clove into a bowl and add a squeeze of lemon to taste, add oil, honey, sea salt, tarragon (fresh herbs if you like.) If necessary, add a little water if the lemon juice is too tart or strong. Pour over salad.

- **ITALIAN DRESSING**

1/4 cup cold pressed olive oil
1 clove garlic
Juiced lemon
Celtic sea salt
1/2 tsp. dried basil/fresh basil leaves
Little pure water.

Crush garlic in a bowl. Add oil, salt, basil, lemon juice, shake and squeeze over salad.

- **PESTO DRESSING**

1 bunch of fresh basil
1/2 cup pine nuts
1/3 cup extra virgin olive oil
Juice of 1 lemon
Celtic sea salt
Grated parmesan cheese/goat's feta cheese/raw cheese
Little pure water.

Wash basil and dry. Place leaves into a blender with the nuts, oil, lemon juice, cheese and salt. Blend until almost smooth. If the dressing is too tart perhaps the lemon is too strong, use a little water to adjust to your taste. Stir a little dressing through pasta with a little parmesan cheese or goat's feta cheese. Refrigerate the rest for later.

- **HOMMUS**

1 cup of chick peas
1/2 cup of tahini
2 cloves of fresh garlic
Chives
Little water
Juice of 1 lemon
Celtic sea salt

Do not use normal table salt. Never use pepper.

Soak fresh chickpeas overnight and drain, then place in blender with tahini, garlic, lemon juice and a pinch of salt. Blend on slow speed until you reach the desired consistency. If it is too thick, use a little pure water to help facilitate blending. Add more lemon juice if desired, to suit your taste. Hummus is great for dipping raw vegetables and if you want to use hummus for a salad dressing dilute it with more lemon juice and or pure water. Garnish with chives. You could also add, freshly grated pumpkin, making pumpkin hummus. Yummy.

I am sure you will have wonderful healthy ideas of your own to try.

All men who have achieved great things
have been great dreamers.
Orison Swett Marden

Every moment is made glorious by the light of love
Rumi

Chapter 11

—Raw/vegan diet for superior health, well being and longevity—

Raw/vegan diets have cured cancer, rheumatoid arthritis, multiple sclerosis, heart disease, lupus, diabetes, asthma, migraines, gangrene, crohn's disease, aids, chronic fatigue syndrome, colitis, hormonal problems, injuries and many more. You could also try it for Parkinson's Disease. What do you have to lose?

A raw/vegan diet has even regenerated bone. It regenerates teeth and the cavities fall out, providing you are drinking green smoothies every day. Some people have their hair grow back to its original color.

It will also reverse your biological clock and make you look many years younger than your chronological years. You will have more energy than you have ever known. No more walking sticks, or walking frames, or aches and pains. This is all caused by inflammation. Once the inflammation has gone, you are pain free.

It's best to consume a couple of shots of wheat grass every day, and live on a living food diet high in sprouts, and greens.

It is imperative that you eat organic food for your optimal health and healing, as non organic food is toxic to your health. The chemical sprays are slowly killing us. Organic food does not cost that much more than non organic food, if you buy from your local organic farmer, or market. Sometimes it's the same price, if not cheaper. I would be very weary of organic food from the supermarket, because you don't know how long it has been stored. Supermarkets store fresh produce for up to 10 months in storage.

DAY ONE—MONDAY

- **BREAKFAST**
- **Green smoothie.**
- **Only use organic food.**

Kale
1 large cut up mango
1 large banana
2 Tablespoons of flaxseed mix (See recipe in recovery diet)
1 & 1/2 glasses of cold pure water
1 Aloe Vera plant gel (optional) (See recipe under the heading, Aloe Vera in body of book)
30 mls organic, cold pressed Coconut oil

Place organic greens, either Kale, Bok Choy, Collard greens, Asian greens, Dandelion, dark lettuce or any other dark leafy greens into a blender until the blender is full, without packing it down. Then add the remaining ingredients and blend until smooth.

Makes about 1 litre/4 cups.

Pour into a glass, and place the remaining into the fridge, and drink throughout the morning. This will keep you going until lunch time, as it's very filling. You can put 2 glasses of water into the blender which will make it not so thick. The fruit is the dominating flavor, and you can hardly taste the greens. It's an amazing way of getting your vital greens into you. You could also take your smoothie to work or to the shops in a cool container as it will last all day without going off.

You can use rock melon, kiwi fruit, or any other fruit you like. However, do not use oranges, mandarins, tangelos, or pineapple as they are too acidic and will cause pain if you have rheumatoid arthritis. If you don't have an inflammatory disease, 1 orange and 2-3 slices of pineapple is nice in the smoothie. Providing it's fresh, and not out of a can.

I make this my morning ritual; the greens give you all the minerals and calcium your body will need. You won't need to take supplements. The fruit provides lots of vitamins. In fact, people who do green smoothies every day, providing you are on a 100% raw food diet, no longer have grey hair. The natural color over the years grows back, and they end up with grey tips until it all grows out. Also, their teeth regenerate and their cavities disappear. Even bone regenerates. You will also be getting your omega 3, 6, & 9s with the flaxseed mix. Again, you won't need omega 3 supplements. That way we kill less sea life, and not upset the eco system. For example, krill oil is made from krill that swim in the Antarctic Ocean providing food for penguins and whales. That food belongs to them, not us. We can get all our vitamins and minerals from plant life, as God/mother nature intended.

- **MORNING TEA**
- **Carrot and apple juice, freshly juiced.**

- **LUNCH**

1 cup organic sprouts
1 sliced tomato
Sliced cucumber
Sliced onion
Cold pressed, extra virgin, (organic)Olive oil/apricot oil/organic, cold pressed coconut oil
Lemon juiced
Celtic sea salt

Your favorite fresh herbs, organically grown.
Use either sunflower Sprouts, broccoli sprouts, radish sprouts, alfalfa sprouts, or any sprouts you like. You could use a bit of each.
In a bowl place all ingredients, squeeze over lemon juice and 1-1/2 capfuls of oil, and sprinkle a little Celtic sea salt.

- **DINNER**
- **Fruit smoothie**

1 cup of mixed berries. Fresh or frozen.
1 large banana
30 mls of coconut oil
¾ glass of pure water
Place all ingredients into a blender and blend, enjoy.

DAY TWO—TUESDAY

- **BREAKFAST**
- **Green smoothie** (see day 1)
- **MORNING TEA**
- **Carrot, celery and apple juice. Freshly juiced.**

- **LUNCH**
- **Carrot and sultana salad**

1 cup of grated organic carrots
Lettuce
1 sliced tomato
Sliced onion
Hand full of sultanas
Lemon juiced
Oil
Celtic sea salt

Place all ingredients into a bowl, squeeze over lemon juice, salt and 1-1/2 caps of oil.

- **DINNER**
- **Raw Soup**

1 glass freshly juiced carrot
1/2 avocado

1 cut up tomato
Pinch Celtic sea salt

　　Place all ingredients into a blender and blend until smooth. Serve into a bowl, or container to take on the run. Yummy.

- **BREAKFAST**
- **Green smoothie**

- **LUNCH**
- **Lettuce roll up**

1 Organic iceberg lettuce leaf
Sprouts
Sliced tomato
Sliced onion
Sliced cucumber
Hummus (See recipe in recovery diet)
Place all ingredients into the lettuce leaf and roll.

- **DINNER**
- **Purple cabbage salad**

1/8-1/4 of purple cabbage thinly sliced, or shredded
1 sliced tomato
Sliced cucumber
Sliced onion

Oil
Lemon juiced
Celtic sea salt

Place all ingredients into a bowl, squeeze over lemon juice, oil and salt.

It is best not to have too many foods at once. Other wise it can compromise your digestive system. If you mix it up a bit, you get all the nutrients you need.

If you want to put a little raw pure unheated honey (yellow box is my favorite) into your dressing with a little fresh garlic, by all means. Do not use minced garlic out of a jar. It has apple cider vinegar in it, and it will exacerbate you pain.

There are other recipes in the recovery diet for salads, juices, dressings and fruit smoothies that you can have. I have just given you a couple of days recipes to give you an idea of what to have on a 100% raw/vegan diet. If you eat only a raw/vegan diet, you should have your health back, in about three—six months. But give it at least a year.

If you go off your diet for any reason, you will/may slow the recovery process and undo the good work you have done.

There are plenty of fancy raw/vegan recipes you can try once you are well. When you are overcoming an illness, it is best to keep it simple.

The recovery diet will also reverse lupus, high blood pressure, and I would even try it for all auto-immune diseases, gastric reflux, constipation, heart disease etc; What do you have to lose?

The raw/vegan diet will reverse multiple sclerosis, cancer, rheumatoid arthritis and just about any disease known to man. Many people have done it.

Conclusion

Perhaps it is now clear to you why I have chosen a natural approach to healing my body of rheumatoid arthritis. In the right environment and with correct nutrition, a natural remission will occur. I do not consider that I have established some sort of precedent with my discoveries and success in curing myself of a supposedly incurable disease for there are many people, especially those suffering from cancer, who have eaten their way to good health. There are thousands of success stories around the world. I am simply one of them. You, too, can be a success story.

If you believe you can, you will. If you believe you can't, you won't. If we have limiting beliefs, our lives will be limited. That is why we need to focus on what we want and take action. This includes creating a supportive environment and making conscious decisions to create what we want in our lives, especially when it comes to enforcing boundaries. If we focus on our old patterns, we will merely create the same kind of life for ourselves. For example, if you focus on the root cause of your problems (significant, traumatic childhood emotional events) you will stay connected to them. If we learn to disconnect from those experiences perhaps the problems will disappear as an issue in your life?

A positive mental attitude is paramount to getting well. Believing in yourself is an integral part of regaining your health. Most of all, you have to *want* to get well. Sometimes it is easier not to change because we see it as just too hard to find that much energy and change can frighten many of us. Sometimes it is easier simply to die, even if it is just to escape our pain. Moreover, some of us are wracked with such emotional pain in addition to the physical pain that a release from it all makes death seem the preferred option. It is your choice and that is respected. Whatever your choice, may divine love and peace be with you. However, if you want to get well, believe in your self and you will find your courage.

When I first started on my road to recovery I had no idea what I was doing or even if success was a possibility. I had no support system except for my young children. I had no family to help me, or a medical practitioner who was interested in guiding me. Nor, did I have a natural health care professional as an adviser simply because I never had the resources. In any event, I did not have any expertise or the understanding of rheumatoid arthritis and its complexities. There was one thing I did know, however, and that was that one way or another, I was going to be free of this dreadful disease. I was also absolutely determined never to give up. The thought of ending up in a nursing home relying on the mercy or not, of others was my primary motivator. It would mean repeating my childhood, by being back in a home again, without any control over my needs.

I tried everything there was. I renounced our Western diet overnight and started to eat more fruit, vegetables, nuts, seeds and salads. I also started saying positive affirmations to myself while in bed every morning and night. As this is when the mind is in the 'alpha state'—most relaxed—it is also its most receptive. (Children up until the age of seven are permanently in the alpha state).

Some of my affirmations were:

> *Thank you God, for my extraordinary health and fitness.*
> *Thank you God, for giving me the opportunity to help my fellow man.*
> *I love my life.*
> *I am now living the life of my dreams.*
> *I am now living my life's purpose.*
> *I now live in health*
> *I feel fantastic.*
> *I have boundless energy.*

Use these or choose your own affirmations but you must make your affirmations in the present tense so that the Universe can bring them into your reality. In other words, they must always say, 'I am, I have' and not 'I will.' I know this works because it works for thousands of people around the world who use affirmations to bring their dreams into reality.

As an example, I gave up smoking on December 8, 1991 by repeatedly saying affirmations. As I inhaled on each cigarette I said, "I am a non smoker." As I blew out the smoke I said, "I am a non smoker." In bed at night and first thing in the morning I affirmed,

"I am a non smoker." I said it over and over, and with each cigarette, until one night six months later, when I was just about to retire to bed, I went to put the cigarettes high up in the cupboard away from the children, my usual automatic ritual. Something inside of me said, "I am a non-smoker" and I threw the cigarettes into the bin.

It was so easy I almost felt guilty. I have not had a cigarette since. "Because I am, a non smoker." That is how powerful the mind is. The mind is more powerful than the body. How you programme yourself is how you will end up. What you think—you will create. That is why it is so important to have a positive mental attitude. It is vital to stay away from negative people who might nullify your positivity.

Toxic relationships are dangerous to our health and if you are in such an association whether it is a spouse, partner, parents, children, relatives, co-workers or friends then it needs to be addressed. "Who you mix with, you become." Don't spend time with people you don't want to be. A harmonious environment is crucial to getting well. We all know that stress is a very big killer. Rheumatoid arthritis is stressful enough without added burdens. Remember it is not only what you are eating, but with whom you are eating.

Once you are on the maintenance diet, if you start to have any pain, then omit any new food that you have introduced and start back on the recovery diet and introduce one new food at a time for a week or two, and see if you have any reaction.

If you start to go back slowly on to Western Diet food, you will suffer the consequences and it will only be a matter of time before RA could return or you develop another disease.

In order to properly cleanse your body of toxins and to stay healthy, you need to stay on the recovery diet for at least twelve months. If you are pain free and in remission by the end of twelve months then go onto the maintenance diet. However, if your pain comes back, take notice of what you are eating and omit that from the menu. If you want to maintain your health, you must start listening to your body because it is always sending us messages. Our bodies are screaming out at us but most of us do not listen, let alone act on them. You will eventually become closely attuned to your body and you will know it better than anyone.

For example, no one knows better than does a mother when something is wrong with her baby. They may not know what is wrong, but know that something is very wrong. Even when doctors are telling them that there is nothing wrong, mothers know intuitively there is, and keep on searching until they find the answers to their concern. This is how you will become with your own body. When you feed your body highly nutritious food and get rid of all the junk you ate previously, your body will speak to you. All you have to do, is listen.

If you are lucky enough to start this diet when you are first diagnosed with this disease, you may be able to prevent the damage to your joints and body before it starts, but no matter how sick, old, or deformed you are it is not too late to help yourself. Do not think for one moment it is too late. It is never too late and do not let anyone tell you it is. When doctors tell their patients they have six months to live with cancer and that they will be dead by Christmas, they are dead by Christmas, simply because they believed what the doctor said. The mind takes over with that belief. The doctor does not mention that diet can help. Some of them rarely give their patients any options.

When you believe what others tell you, you are giving away your power and in doing that, they own you. Learn to believe in yourself because you are all you have. Believe you can do this and believe you will be well again. Put it up to the Universe and ask for help, talk to your God. Use positive affirmations every day and become a positive thinker, even on your worst day, sitting in your chair that you cannot get out of, tell yourself again and again, "I am in perfect health." Visualize yourself walking, laughing and enjoying life pain free. You will see it, when you believe it, it is that simple.

Rise up out of your chair—at least mentally to begin with—and reach out for yourself. Reach for the person deep inside of you and give your life a purpose. We were not meant to live in poverty and ill health. We are meant to know the joys of life—to share our knowledge and our gifts; to share love and kindness. To share the magic that life can offer us, and to share that magic with those who need it most of all. First, though, we need it ourselves in order to give to others. Ask God for help, and just know and believe you can do this. If you do not believe in God, then believe in the power of the Universe, or at least believe in yourself, but believe in something. Do not give up on yourself for you owe it to yourself to take the chance to be the person you were meant to be. You are on this earth for a reason. You are important and you matter, and your life does have meaning. Your life does have a purpose, just believe in yourself and know that you, too, can be healthy. Remember,

God does not make mistakes; you are here for a purpose. I believe in you and send you divine love and peace every day. I am thinking of you and your suffering. You are in my prayers.

Health has become my passion. I live and breathe it every day and I choose never to go back on Western diet food simply because it no longer appeals to me. I have become addicted to healthy food, just the way people become addicted to high fat foods, sugar, alcohol, cigarettes and additives. I love feeling healthy, I love feeling light and energetic. I love having freedom from rheumatoid arthritis.

I no longer lay in my bed at night unable to roll over or move because of the swelling and pain in my shoulders and knees. I no longer rely on my children to dress me, feed me, and place me on the toilet bowl. For me it is over, it is just a blur. Now I can do these things for myself. I have my mobility back, I have my dignity back and yes, I have my life back. I have control again and as a result, I am now a different person.

I have not emerged unscathed from my battle with rheumatoid arthritis. I may never be able to play tennis again. I may not be able to play contact sport again, I have to admit, I am working on it. I never give up. But I can walk 25 kilometers a week and more if I had the time. To look at me you would not know I had ever been afflicted with rheumatoid arthritis. I look healthy, I look fit and I am very fit on the inside. I do not take medication for anything. Most people my age are on medication for some type of disease—for instance, diabetes, obesity, high blood pressure, angina, heart disease, stroke, some form of arthritis and even cancer.

For this reason I continue to keep myself healthy and that is why I walk five kilometers, five or six days a week. I eat a high raw diet; this includes a dark green leafy vegetable smoothies and salad every day. Living on the Gold Coast in Queensland, the warm climate allows me to eat a high raw diet. I have eaten different food at Christmas sometimes, perhaps for two or three days or one meal on special occasions such as birthdays, simply because I am healthy enough to do this. Sometimes I break out and have what ever I want. When I do this, it makes me appreciate my healthy food as I have become addicted to it. Do not do this on the recovery diet. However, two or three days, is all I can tolerate, because I cannot stand the way I feel after wards. I love the feeling of a fresh crisp salad in my mouth; I love knowing how nutritious it is and the good it is doing for my body.

Incidentally, my friends affectionately call me the "Health Guru" because they know how passionate I am about my health and health in general. They are amazed at how disciplined I am but for me it is simple. I have just learned to love health and anything to do with health. I no longer live to eat. I eat to live. I read everything I can on diet and disease. I have learned to appreciate my well-being simply because I know what it feels like to be chronically ill. I have been given a second chance and I am not going to do anything to jeopardize it.

According to Louise L. Hay, author of "You can heal your life" our emotional pain and suffering is the cause of disease. She goes on to say that arthritis is caused by "feeling unloved, criticism and resentment." I was unloved, criticized and I resented the perpetrators who assaulted me. If this is true then is it any wonder I developed rheumatoid arthritis. I do believe that in conjunction with a high fat diet and poor eating habits, emotions definitely play a significant role in our health and well-being. Any emotional trauma is stressful and stress can kill.

In order to heal my body I first had to learn to love myself and know that I was okay regardless of what other people did to me in the past, or what they thought of me. I had to start taking care of me, physically, emotionally, mentally and spiritually. And that meant reclaiming my body, my health and my life and to take back control over my own emotions, life and health. I am now in charge, I am now in control and it is up to me to take stock of my emotions and take back my power. This means I am responsible and accountable for my own health, including the food that I choose to put into my body.

Moreover, the healthy food that I choose to put into my body will make me well. You, too, can do this, I know you can, because every moment is precious and every moment is your life. Do this in spite of your emotional pain, in spite of your negators. As Oprah Winfrey once said, "Use your emotional pain to drive you to success." Believe me, it can be done. Many people have done it and many people have cured themselves of cancer and other diseases, too. I know if you just give yourself a chance and start to believe in you again you will be able to do anything. No matter what the odds, anything is possible. There is hope for everybody in this world no matter how sick you may be. Just believe you can, that is all you have to do. Look at the sick person you are and think about the person you ought to be.

I know some of you have burdens known only to yourselves and I know how this illness can strip away from us our self-definition, but where there is life, there is hope. Reclaim your life. Reclaim your health for if we find one small excuse not to follow through, we will soon find a hundred and be the same as we were before. Do not give up on yourself. If you give up on you, then what do you have left? Use any reason there is to help yourself to regain your health. Think about the goals and dreams you once believed in before you were struck down with RA. Learn to dream again. Even on only the wisp of hope, you *can* dream. You can live these dreams again and make them come into fruition. You can manifest your dreams into your reality. And if you believe in your dreams, you give them life. Believe in *you* once again and the Universe will believe in you too.

Do not believe what the doctors tell you about RA being incurable. *Results* are what count. Some doctors do not believe diet can cure anything. They only believe what is under a microscope. They support the medicine, not the immune system, which God gave us in his genius. They cannot even save themselves because they do not believe they can. Some medical experts are so pre-occupied with their own expertise they impose it on their patients and fail to notice what their patients want. What I want is a healthy body with a long quality of life. And I do not want rheumatoid arthritis. And I certainly do not want medication that will numb my brain into a stupor while I die a slow agonizing death. I wanted support from my doctors to help me to achieve health but it was never forthcoming. All I got was condescension and bullying because I refused to take the drugs; I believed there had to be a way other than chemical drugs with shocking side effects that create other diseases.

I had to believe in me in order to do what I have achieved. If I was not born with RA then why do I have to have it now? I found my strength and courage and believed in me when others did not. I have also reached a point in my life where I don't care what other people think of me. What is important is what I think of me. I think I am Okay. You are too. To all the sufferers out there, I believe in you, and I will pray for you to find your courage, your self worth, your strength and your faith in yourself once again. After all, you are human beings and I believe in humanity. The greatest test of all is to believe in yourself when others around you do not. Dig deep down into the deepest recess of your pain and believe that you can do anything.

I believed I could cure myself and write this book even though it took me one year to get through the first chapter because I did not want to remember how it was. I understand no matter how bad things have been, or how bad things are now in your life, you can achieve anything you want to. If you give yourself half a chance; you can do anything. The power of positive thinking will take you anywhere you want to go. Just know it, live it, feel it and believe it. Do not give up on yourself; you are all you have.

My life is too precious; my body is too precious to poison it everyday with Western diet food, toxic medications, and toxic relationships. My organs work to perfection without me even knowing, the blood pumps through my arteries and veins and I do not even feel it. My heart beats to keep me alive and I am not even aware of it. All this I have learned to appreciate. I have learned that my body needs proper nutrition in order to work properly, in order to keep me healthy. Knowing what I now know about health and well-being, I will not allow it to be jeopardized.

When we stray too far from nature, we will pay the consequences. It is just a matter of time and you can almost pick your disease. There are plenty out there from which to choose. And if you believe that you will die of heart disease and expect it in your fifties because your parents died of it, then more than likely you will, simply because you believe you will and you plant that seed and in doing so bring your greatest fear to reality. However if you live on highly nutritious food, and not Western diet food you will dramatically decrease your chances of premature death. As Dr Mehmet C, Oz states, it's choice of food that kills us, not genetics. If you believe you will develop rheumatoid arthritis and expect it to happen because it is in the family then more than likely you will. Again, living a healthy lifestyle and exercise may reduce your risks. What you fear you will bring about.

If you believe you can, you will. If you believe you can't, you won't. What you think you are and what you believe you create; what you eat today walks and talks tomorrow. I believe I am healthy and that I will live a long healthy life. I believe I will never end up in a nursing home. For me that would be like being back in the orphanage with other people in control of me and the possibility that once again my needs would not be met. I refuse to be at the mercy of others. Some people unfortunately, see you as easy prey when you are chronically ill, and treat you as a victim. I will not be a victim; it is too draining, too demoralizing and too negative.

Although I eat very healthy food my children, however, do not eat what I eat. It is too strict for them and so I cook normal Western food with emphasis on fruit, salads and vegetables. Now they are in their twenties, they love their junk food like other young people their age and because they have their own money, I cannot control what they eat. I would not force my eating habits on anyone especially my children, but should they become sick in the future, hopefully, they will remember what I did and they will allow me to help them.

As far as my emotions are concerned, I have worked through a lot of my issues. I sometimes think about mother and ponder on how it all could have been. I think about all the opportunities she missed in loving me and the opportunities I missed in being loved. My biggest regret is that I was never anyone's little girl. I was never significant, meaningful or special. But she has been gone a long time now, and I have learned to move on to lead the best possible life I can with what I know and what I have learned. I made a conscious decision to disconnect myself from my past traumatic events that happened to me, simply because they weigh me down and prevent me from moving on and having a happy life. They prevent me from being the person I want to be. From being the person I choose to be. Carrying around that kind of emotional baggage is debilitating and limiting. It just keeps you in the misery re-living it over and over until you become an emotional cripple. When we carry around our negative emotions that is all we will attract in our lives. If we are loaded down with misery, how can we attract happiness or anything worthwhile? Worrying about the past or the future will only re-enforce the problem to continue. Worry is a waste of time and emotions, it causes ill health. Focusing on the negative will only re-enforce it into your life. This is why it is imperative to focus on the positive. I make a point never to focus on a problem. I focus only on the solution. You will be surprised how problems just disappear.

It took a lot for me to move on because my history was who I was. It was the evidence of my existence. It was familiar. It was comfortable. It was my friend. It was *my* life. Now I choose a different life for myself because I am strong. I am who I am. I am no longer the little girl who, when frightened by her world retreats to a locker. Furthermore, I have developed a tremendous amount of self respect. Therefore, I choose to be free of the past. Free of my memories. Free of toxic relationships. Free of rheumatoid arthritis. Free to forgive my mother. "Mum, if you are watching over me, I forgive you and I love you. I always have." I am yet to meet that special someone in my life, someone who is kind and tender. I guess we spend most of our lives searching for love and purpose. Some of us find it. I live in hope. You never know if you believe.

Knowing that "man cannot live by bread alone" I try to lead a balanced and stress free life. This is why it is so important to address any negative relationships you may have and to keep any stresses in your life to a minimum. If you do not, rheumatoid arthritis will exact a heavy toll on the quality of that life.

I send you divine love and peace and wish you excellent health, courage and good luck in this, and in all your endeavors. Because of my love and compassion for humanity my desire is to make a difference in this world. If I have helped you to help yourself, then I have made a difference. I welcome your feedback and would love to hear from you about your progress.

I wish you all a wonderful and pain free life. I wish you freedom from your physical and emotional pain. God bless you. You deserve it. *www.ffra.com*

THE END

Nothing splendid has ever been achieved except by those who dared believe that something inside them was superior to circumstance

Bruce Barton

Great spirits have always encountered violent opposition from mediocre minds.

Albert Einstein

Dear (to whom it may concern) I won't be needing your help today, love God.

anonymous

Bibliography

Brooks, and Dortok. eds. *Proceedings of the Royal Society of Medicine Natural Health*. 1992.

Carper, Jean. *Food Your Miracle Medicine.* How Food Can Prevent & Treat Over 100 Symptoms & Problems. London: Simon & Schuster, 1995.

Hay, Louise L. *You Can Heal Your Life*. NSW: Specialist Publications, 1987.

Holzapfel, Cynthia and Laura. *Coconut Oil* for Health and Beauty. USA: Book Publishing Company, 2003.

Horne, Ross. *The Health Revolution*. NSW: Happy Landings, 1981.

Jensen, Bernard. *Tissue Cleansing Through Bowel Management*. From the Simple to the Ultimate. California: Bernard Jensen, 1981.

Lond, William K. *Mind & Body.* 1969.

Lorand, Arnold. *Old Age Deferred.* 1910.

Lyman, Howard F. *Mad Cowboy.* Plain Truth from The Cattle Rancher Who Won't Eat Meat. New York: Simon & Schuster Inc, 1998.

Mendelsohn, Robert S. *Confessions of a Medical Heretic*. Chicago: Contemporary Books, 1979.

Oz, Mehmet C. *You, the owner's manual* USA: Alliance Publishing, 2005.

Vance, Judi. *Beauty to Die For*. The Cosmetic Consequence. Canada: Promotion Publishing, 1998.